Neuropathy Nutrition Protocol for Seniors

A Science-Backed Anti-Inflammatory System for Managing Nerve Pain from Shingles, Diabetes, and Age-Related Nerve Damage - With Nerve-Supporting Food Science, 65 Easy Recipes, and a 28-Day Recovery Plan

Disclaimer

This guide is provided for informational and educational purposes only and should not be interpreted as medical, nutritional, or professional advice. The author is not a licensed physician, nurse, dietitian, or mental health provider. Reading this guide does not establish a patient-provider relationship of any kind.

Always seek the guidance of a qualified healthcare professional before starting, changing, or discontinuing any supplement, diet, or lifestyle program. If you are pregnant, breastfeeding, managing a chronic medical condition, or taking prescription medications, consult your physician or pharmacist before considering any product mentioned in this guide.

The author and publisher make no representations or warranties regarding accuracy, applicability, fitness, or completeness of the information contained herein. While every effort has been made to ensure scientific accuracy and currency, medical knowledge and research evolve continually. Readers are responsible for verifying information and making decisions in consultation with licensed professionals.

Use of this guide and any information contained within it is at your own risk. The author and publisher disclaim all liability for any loss, injury, or adverse outcome that may result from the use or misuse of this material.

No supplement, diet, or practice discussed in this text is intended to diagnose, treat, cure, or prevent any disease. No outcomes or benefits are guaranteed.

Product names, supplement formulations, diet frameworks, and trademarks mentioned are the property of their respective owners and are used for identification only. Any images or illustrations that appear in related materials are licensed stock or educational placeholders.

Table of Contents

Introduction

A senior's day can so often be shaped by sensations others take for granted: a tingling foot on the floor, numbness in the hands, or a shot of pain after standing up. These challenges, rooted in nerve damage, impact not only comfort but also balance, independence, and quality of life. For many older adults, the source may be diabetes, shingles, medication side effects, age-related declines, or even missed nutrients. Living with neuropathy is as much about managing daily discomfort as it is about preserving the freedoms of movement, restful sleep, and confidence.

The reality is that when peripheral neuropathy remains unaddressed, its effects reach far beyond tingling or aches. Problems with nerve signaling can gradually sap mobility, erode balance, disturb sleep, and make routine activities feel daunting. This can lead to a loss of confidence, hesitancy to walk in unfamiliar places, reluctance to cook, even avoidance of outings for fear of falls or fatigue. The risk of diminished independence becomes real, underscoring why purposeful self-care is vital at any age but especially in later years.

Hope lives in the details of daily habits. While no plan can reverse severe nerve damage or replace medical care, purposeful nutrition and lifestyle strategies can meaningfully slow nerve decline, support healing, decrease discomfort, and help restore ease in daily life. Science recognizes that the foods you choose influence inflammation, nerve nutrition, blood flow, and recovery speed. Each meal is an opportunity to supply the body with not only calories, but also the building blocks required for nerve health and repair.

While many guides promise miracle cures or pitch the latest supplement, this resource takes a grounded, practical, and sustainable approach. You won't find dramatic claims or discouraging technical jargon here. Instead, you'll find clear explanations and hands-on strategies focused exclusively on lifestyle, food, and supportive routines for those living with neuropathy. The guidance presented helps you reduce symptoms, protect nerve function, and build confidence not by replacing medication, but by strengthening the foundation for whole-body wellness. Pharmaceutical treatments, diagnostic tests, and medical interventions lie outside this book's scope; for those, continued partnership with your healthcare provider remains vital.

In this guide, you will discover:

- The science behind nerve health in older adults including how nerves become damaged and the most significant contributors to ongoing symptoms.
- Detailed breakdowns of which foods, nutrients, and dietary habits can ease neuropathic discomfort or slow its progression.
- Easy-to-understand meal planning systems, showing how to prioritize and combine anti-inflammatory ingredients for both enjoyment and function.
- A phased 28-day nutrition plan tailored specifically for seniors, with practical guidance for adjusting routines, tracking results, and responding to changing symptoms.

- Sixty-five carefully designed recipes involving breakfasts, lunches, dinners, snacks, and smoothies, all developed to deliver the most nerve-supportive nutrition possible.
- Movement adaptations, kitchen tips, and symptom tracking tools made for those living with sensory changes, weaker grip, or limited vision.
- Common questions answered with actionable advice for everyday obstacles faced by seniors living with neuropathy.

The benefits of nutrition are cumulative and best realized with steady, consistent changes rather than quick fixes or restrictive rules. This guide walks beside you meal by meal, week by week as you discover a new sense of control over symptom management and wellbeing.

If you have questions, complex conditions, or changing symptoms while following this protocol, involve your physician or a registered dietitian who knows your history. Safe progress is steady and individualized.

With patience, knowledge, and the right toolkit, it is possible to reclaim greater ease and resilience despite neuropathy. This journey is about nourishing both nerves and confidence, and it begins with the choices you make each day.

Understanding Neuropathy in Older Adults

Across the landscape of age-related health, neuropathy stands out for the way it quietly disrupts well-being, sometimes creeping in with subtle tingling, at other times arriving with sharper pain or profound numbness. It is not a single disease, but a result of many strands of nerve injury woven together by life's circumstances: a case of longstanding diabetes, the wake of a shingles outbreak, nutritional deficits, reactions to medication, or the slow shifts that naturally occur with age. For older adults, deciphering these causes is central to reclaiming comfort, mobility, and confidence in daily life.

Categories of Non-Traumatic Nerve Damage

Neuropathy in seniors rarely comes from obvious injuries. Instead, it develops through more subtle, chronic processes often affecting the hands and feet first. **Among non-traumatic types, five categories stand out:**

1. **Diabetic Neuropathy:** Persistently high blood sugar damages the delicate fibers in peripheral nerves over months and years. Diabetes is a leading reason older adults develop neuropathy, with symptoms intensifying when blood glucose

is less well-controlled. This form not only causes discomfort, but also raises the risk for ulcers, infections, and falls.

2. **Post-shingles (Postherpetic Neuralgia):** After an outbreak of shingles, some individuals—especially those over 60 develop lingering nerve pain in the affected skin areas. This burning or electric shock-like sensation can persist long after the rash fades, interfering with comfort, clothing choices, and sleep.
3. **Age-Related Changes:** The nervous system naturally changes with advancing age. Nerves become less efficient at transmitting signals, circulation may decline, and the body's ability to repair minor damage drops. Sometimes, there is no single "trigger" but rather a gradual loss of function often first felt as numbness or tingling in the toes or fingers.
4. **Medication-Induced Neuropathy:** Certain drugs prescribed for other conditions can inadvertently injure nerves, especially when more than one medication is used at the same time a situation called polypharmacy. Older adults with complex medication regimens may be especially susceptible.
5. **Nutrition-Deficiency Neuropathy:** Some vitamin and mineral deficiencies can diminish nerve health. Most commonly, deficits in B-vitamins (especially B12), vitamin E, and minerals like magnesium may arise when diets lack variety, appetite wanes, or absorption is impaired by other illnesses or medications.

Each type may appear alone or in combination, making it essential to identify root causes with your medical team. Importantly, no single profile fits every older adult, and symptoms can blur across types. For instance, diabetes and nutritional gaps often go hand-in-hand, while medications might exacerbate existing age-related vulnerabilities.

Common Sensory Symptoms, Signaling Patterns, and Safety-Risks in Seniors

Peripheral neuropathy often begins with subtle changes in sensation—sometimes dismissed as "just getting older." Early recognition of patterns can help prevent serious complications:

- Tingling ("pins and needles"), burning, or prickling in the feet or hands, which may worsen at night or after prolonged sitting.
- Numbness or reduced ability to feel temperature, which can make it difficult to detect blisters, burns, or cuts.
- Sharp, stabbing, or electric shock-like pains, sometimes shooting suddenly or triggered by touch or pressure.
- Increased sensitivity where even gentle touch or light pressure causes disproportionate discomfort.
- Weakness or sense of heaviness, making walking or grasping objects more challenging.
- Changes in temperature perception, causing misjudgment of water heat, heating pads, or outdoor cold.

Because neuropathy damages the nerves responsible for sensing pain or injury, these symptoms create specific risks in later life. The most common safety concerns include:

- Higher likelihood of falls due to unsteadiness, weak ankle muscles, or numbness.
- Reduced awareness of minor injuries, leading to wounds or infections, particularly on the feet where visual checks are difficult.
- Invisible burns from hot water, stoves, or heating appliances when sensory feedback is impaired.
- Worsened balance, which may lead to a hesitancy to move or exercise, contributing to muscle loss and reduced circulation.

For seniors living alone, or for those managing existing vision or mobility challenges, these safety issues call for heightened vigilance and for establishing supportive routines to check skin regularly, maintain safe home environments, and seek prompt care for new or unexplained symptoms.

Nerve Damage Progression Timeline: How Underlying Causes Unfold

Visualizing the progression of neuropathy helps clarify why timely nutrition and lifestyle changes matter. Here, a conceptual timeline demonstrates typical patterns for each major cause. Although individual experiences will differ, understanding these "trajectories" can anchor expectations and guide prevention efforts.

1. **Diabetic Neuropathy**
   - Initial Stage (Months to Years): Subtle tingling or numbness appears in the toes or fingertips.
   - Mid-Stage: Persistent burning, hypersensitivity, and night-time pain develop. Blood sugar spikes accelerate further damage.

- o Advanced Stage: Loss of sensation, muscle weakness, frequent foot injuries, and deep ulcers may occur if blood sugar remains uncontrolled.

2. **Post-Shingles Neuralgia**
   - o Acute Phase: Shingles rash with pain, usually resolving in weeks.
   - o Subacute: In approximately 1 in 5 older adults, severe nerve pain persists for months post-rash.
   - o Chronic: In some cases, pain endures for years, often worsened by stress or poor nutrition.
3. **Age-Related Neuropathy**
   - o Subtle Onset (Years): Gradual, patchy numbness or tingling surfaces, often dismissed as "just aging."
   - o Worsening Over Time: Sensory loss extends; walking or dexterity difficulties may follow, especially if inactivity or other chronic illnesses are involved.
4. **Medication-Induced Neuropathy**
   - o Onset: Symptoms can begin weeks to months after starting a new medication, or when dose increases.
   - o Progression: Persisting exposure worsens nerve dysfunction, but early identification and discontinuation can sometimes halt or reverse symptoms.
5. **Nutritional Deficiency Neuropathy**
   - o Insidious Beginning: Mild tingling or numbness, fatigue, and unsteadiness start quietly, especially if diet remains restricted.
   - o Progressive Worsening: More pronounced weakness, balance problems, and cognitive changes manifest without correction of deficiencies.

In each category, catching early warning signs rather than waiting for "big problems" is crucial for maintaining function, safety, and overall quality of life. Timely attention to diet, blood sugar, and routine screening can slow or even partially reverse early symptoms for some individuals.

Factors Making Seniors Uniquely Vulnerable to Neuropathy Worsening

Why are older adults at especially high risk for neuropathy progression? Several biological and practical realities intersect to raise vulnerability:

- **Slower Healing:** Age-related declines in cell repair make it more difficult for nerves to bounce back from injury. This means that any minor damage whether from blood sugar spikes, virus reactivation, or small wounds takes longer to heal, increasing the risk for progression and complications.
- **Polypharmacy:** Many seniors use multiple medications to manage chronic illnesses. Some of these drugs may damage nerves, interact with each other to amplify side effects, or block the absorption of critical vitamins and minerals. When numerous medications are involved, pinpointing the source of neuropathy or making safe changes can be complicated.
- **Weakened Circulation:** The small blood vessels that keep nerves oxygenated tend to narrow with age, especially with longstanding diabetes or cardiovascular disease. Poor blood flow further impairs the delivery of nutrients required for nerves to function and repair.

- **Reduced Mobility:** Discomfort from neuropathy often discourages physical activity, yet inactivity itself can worsen nerve symptoms, reduce joint flexibility, and slow healing.
- **Nutritional Shortfalls:** Appetite changes, dental issues, economic constraints, and occasional difficulty preparing meals can lead older adults toward more restricted, less diverse diets. Over time, this raises the risk for deficiencies in nerve-critical nutrients.
- **Heightened Injury Risk:** Decreased sensation in the feet or hands means minor cuts, blisters, or burns may go unnoticed, resulting in infections or chronic wounds more easily missed if vision is also impaired.

These vulnerabilities do not mean that decline is inevitable, but rather highlight where targeted, proactive strategies like those in this guide can offer the greatest benefit. Addressing each factor through diet, environment updates, and close coordination with healthcare professionals becomes a powerful tool for prevention and symptom relief.

Safe Communication Framework: Sharing Neuropathy Symptoms, Dietary Shifts, and Supplements with Healthcare Teams

A key part of effective neuropathy management lies in coordinated communication both clear and timely between seniors, their family members, and their healthcare providers. The following framework supports productive dialogue about symptoms, diet changes, and supplement use:

1. **Be Precise and Consistent in Reporting Symptoms:** Keep a simple log of when symptoms began, what they feel like (for example, location, intensity, triggers, and timing), and whether they are changing over time. Noting when discomfort spikes such as after certain activities, meals, or at night—helps medical providers pinpoint underlying factors and assess risk patterns more accurately.
2. **Communicate Dietary Shifts and Supplement Use:** Any change in diet especially if it involves new foods, reduced sodium, or supplements like B-vitamins and magnesium should be communicated with healthcare teams. This is especially relevant for older adults managing diabetes, heart disease, or on medications that can interact with certain nutrients. By sharing updated meal habits or supplement lists during check-ups, providers can look for potential interactions, adjust prescriptions, and order blood tests to monitor nutrient levels where needed.
3. **Address Medication and Side Effects:** If neuropathy symptoms appear or change after starting, stopping, or increasing a medication, bring this up at your earliest convenience. It is common for multiple medications to interact in ways that affect nerve function. Rather than stopping or changing any medicine on your own, work with your care team to review all prescriptions regularly.
4. **Prepare Questions in Advance:** Writing down questions before visits whether about uncomfortable sensations, nutritional concerns, or safe exercise is practical and empowers seniors to have their priorities addressed. Consider

bringing a trusted friend or family member to take notes or help communicate issues if needed.

5. **Engage in Ongoing Collaboration:** Healthcare is most effective when it's a two-way conversation. Providers can help adjust recommendations, test for underlying causes, or refer to specialists, but only when equipped with the most up-to-date information about symptoms and lifestyle habits. Don't hesitate to ask for detailed explanations about test results, or how dietary suggestions fit alongside prescribed treatments.

This coordinated approach prevents the well-documented pitfalls of isolated self-care or communication gaps. It becomes especially urgent when considering the overlap between chronic conditions common in older adults, like diabetes, hypertension, and digestive disorder all of which impact nerve health through direct or indirect means.

Avoiding Pitfalls When Adjusting Diet or Supplements

An open discussion is also essential before making changes to what or how you eat. Older adults with neuropathy may have comorbidities or medication regimens that affect how nutrients are absorbed or processed.

For example, using a multivitamin or B12 supplement might seem like an easy solution for numbness until it is discovered that a medication lowers absorption or a kidney condition alters safe dosing thresholds. Providers can help you customize choices to your personal health profile, monitor blood values, or suggest specialist referrals when symptoms persist despite your best efforts.

In addition, choosing to exclude certain foods whether to manage blood sugar, lower sodium, or alleviate sensitivity to ingredients should be discussed rather than managed in isolation. Dietary patterns that work for one condition may be too restrictive for another, so expert guidance ensures that all needs are balanced.

Cultivating a Support System

Living with neuropathy often brings emotional and practical hurdles. Shared routines like meal preparation, skin checks, guided exercise, or symptom tracking are easier and safer when done in partnership with caregivers, friends, or family members. Regular communication keeps loved ones aware of changing needs, provides accountability to new habits, and ensures that no sign of complication is missed unnecessarily.

Bringing caregivers and loved ones into the conversation with healthcare providers supports seamless, all-around care and lifts the burden from any one individual. This team-centered approach is especially meaningful for seniors navigating complex medical landscapes or adapting to new diagnoses later in life.

Aging brings plenty of uncertainties, but understanding neuropathy's causes, risks, and progression removes much of its mystery and anxiety. By differentiating diabetic, post-shingles, medication-induced, age-related, and deficiency-driven nerve symptoms, seniors and their caregivers can build vigilance and resilience to better prevent complications, preserve independence, and maintain quality of life.

Equipped with a clear overview of symptom patterns, progression timelines, and the value of coordinated care, you're ready to adopt the proactive dietary and lifestyle strategies outlined in the coming chapters. With the right information and a spirit of teamwork, the changing landscape of nerves in older age can be navigated with confidence, grace, and a renewed sense of control.

Nerve Health Foundations—Core Nutrients and Mechanisms

When considering how to maintain nerve health in older adulthood, the focus often lands on symptom management or prescription regimens. Beneath the surface, what truly determines the long-term resilience of your nerves is a daily accumulation of nutritional and metabolic choices shaping not just how nerves function, but whether they can withstand stress, repair themselves, and continue supporting sensation and movement.

Rather than a distant, theoretical goal, nerve vitality emerges from fundamental processes taking place in every meal, sip, and supplement decision. To create a practical foundation for your recovery toolkit, this chapter unpacks the essential nutrients, biological roadblocks, and absorption realities shaping nerve health for seniors. Rather than a static list of vitamins, think of these elements as gears in a complex engine each contributing uniquely to how nerves transmit messages, withstand damage, and potentially heal.

The Core Nutrients Driving Nerve Structure and Repair

At the cellular level, nerve cells are among the most metabolically active and delicate structures in the human body. Their ability to transmit information, relay pain or temperature, and recover from injury depends on a precise supply of macro- and micronutrients.

Many older adults have heard about B12 in relation to nerves, but nerve health is a team effort involving multiple nutrients working together:

- **B Vitamins:** Among the B vitamins, B1 (thiamine), B6 (pyridoxine), and B12 (cobalamin) rank as the most critical for everything from energy metabolism inside nerves to myelin sheath maintenance (the fatty layer insulating nerve fibers). In people with diabetes or those over 60, deficiencies in these vitamins are surprisingly common and can directly cause or worsen neuropathic symptoms. Supplementation may be recommended if dietary intake or absorption is insufficient, but regular food sources such as leafy greens, whole grains, eggs, dairy, seafood, and fortified cereals play a key role in prevention.
- **Magnesium:** This mineral is fundamental for the conduction of electrical signals along nerves. It not only helps transmit messages but also plays a stress-buffering role: low levels are associated with muscle cramps, nerve irritability, and sensitivity to pain. Magnesium-rich choices include nuts, seeds, legumes, whole grains, and some leafy vegetables.

- **Omega-3 Fatty Acids:** Unlike saturated fats, omega-3s reduce inflammation and help fine blood vessels supply oxygen and nourishment to delicate peripheral nerves. Seniors often need to boost their intake intentionally, as typical diets can fall short. Sources include salmon, sardines, mackerel, walnuts, flaxseeds, chia seeds, and fish oil.
- **Alpha-Lipoic Acid:** While not required in large quantities in the diet, this antioxidant appears to have special benefits in preventing and treating nerve damage in diabetes. It reduces oxidative stress within nerves and may slow disease progression. Some practitioners recommend supplementing it for those with diabetic neuropathy, but it also occurs naturally in spinach, broccoli, and organ meats.
- **Additional Supportive Nutrients:** Vitamins D and E, zinc, and selenium all contribute to nerve membrane integrity, antioxidant defense, and overall repair processes. Fiber (from plant foods) also indirectly supports nerves by stabilizing blood sugar and improving gut health, which in turn enhances absorption of other nutrients critical to nerve function.

What emerges is not a single "magic bullet," but a matrix of vitamins, minerals, and healthy fats consistently present in balanced, minimally processed whole foods. For many older adults, simply eating a wider variety of these foods rather than relying solely on supplements proves protective against slow, cumulative nerve loss.

How Blood Sugar, Inflammation, and Nutritional Gaps Disrupt Nerve Signaling

While nutrition provides construction materials for building and repairing nerve tissue, several invisible forces threaten to undermine this foundation. Among the most damaging are poorly regulated blood sugar, chronic low-grade inflammation, and subtle but crucial nutrient shortfalls. The mechanisms behind these influences reveal why every meal and ingredient choice matters for seniors:

- **High Blood Sugar:** When glucose consistently stays above normal, as in diabetes or pre-diabetes, the surplus sugars physically attach to nerve proteins in a process called glycation. This distorts nerve structure, slows signal speed, and accelerates the loss of sensation and pain control. Over time, frequent spikes (often triggered by high-carb, high-sugar meals) cause direct fiber injury and eventually cell death. Seniors are especially prone to these effects, since insulin sensitivity and sometimes appetite cues decline with age.
- **Chronic Inflammation:** Repeated activation of the body's inflammation system, whether from processed foods, infection, stress, or trauma, contributes to nerve swelling and gradual breakdown. Inflammation restricts blood flow to the periphery, starves nerves of oxygen and nutrients, and triggers the release of damaging free radicals. Diets with excess trans fats, saturated fats, and processed meats fuel this cycle, while anti-inflammatory foods (like fatty fish, green vegetables, berries, turmeric, and ginger) counteract it.

- **Nutritional Gaps:** Subclinical deficiencies particularly in B vitamins, vitamin D, and magnesium block both the formation of myelin (the insulating layer) and the production of the chemicals nerves use to transmit messages. These deficiencies are particularly insidious in older adults: they may cause vague symptoms early on, but quietly accumulate damage over the years. Medications, low appetite, impaired chewing, and digestive changes in later life all conspire to make these gaps more likely and less obvious.

What makes these mechanisms particularly concerning is their tendency to overlap and reinforce each other. High blood sugar worsens inflammation; inflammation impairs absorption; malnutrition leaves nerves vulnerable to both. The take-home message is that targeting only one issue often yields incomplete results. Instead, the steady correction of diet, hydration, and supplementation can put a brake on nerve decline and sometimes help restore lost function.

Quick-Reference Food Sources for Nerve-Supportive Nutrients

A nutritious meal plan for nerve health does not require exotic or hard-to-find products. Rather, common foods chosen well and rotated regularly meet most seniors' needs if prepared and consumed consistently:

B-Vitamins:

- **B1 (thiamine):** Whole grains (brown rice, oats), legumes, nuts, pork, sunflower seeds
- **B6 (pyridoxine):** Chickpeas, chicken, tuna, potatoes, bananas
- **B12 (cobalamin):** Fish, dairy, eggs, fortified plant-based milks and cereals

Magnesium:

- Pumpkin seeds, almonds, spinach, black beans, quinoa, artichokes

Omega-3 Fatty Acids:

- Salmon, mackerel, sardines, chia seeds, flaxseed, walnuts

Alpha-Lipoic Acid:

- Spinach, broccoli, tomatoes, organ meats (liver, kidney)

Vitamin D:

- Egg yolks, fortified dairy and plant drinks, sunlight exposure, salmon

Vitamin E:

- Sunflower seeds, almonds, hazelnuts, avocado, spinach

Trace Minerals (Zinc, Selenium):

- Shellfish (especially oysters), beef, pumpkin seeds, chickpeas, mushrooms

Fiber:

- Leafy greens (kale, chard, collard), berries, sweet potatoes, lentils, oats

Anti-Inflammatory Herbs/Spices:

- Turmeric, ginger, garlic, cinnamon

Among fruits and vegetables, variety remains more powerful than fixation on any single item. Berries, citrus, and colored produce deliver key antioxidants, while green leafy vegetables help regulate immunity and inflammation. A sample "nerve wellness day" might begin with eggs and spinach, include a lentil salad for lunch, snack on nuts, and feature a salmon-and-broccoli dinner. This pattern can be flexibly tailored to taste, budget, and chewing or digestion needs.

Safe and Effective Supplementation: Evidence, Dosing, and Interactions for Seniors

Given the unique vulnerability of seniors to gaps in B vitamins, magnesium, and omega-3s, supplements may seem like a quick solution. However, their use demands accuracy, caution, and continuous coordination with healthcare providers.

Evidence supports the following supplements for nerve health:

- **B-Vitamin Complex:** Especially for those with limited dietary intake, diagnosed deficiencies, or conditions such as diabetes that elevate requirements. Standard doses (for adults 60+) often match or slightly exceed general adult recommendations, but individual tailoring based on lab work is safest. High-dose B6 can cause nerve problems if abused, so combined supplements or single B6-only products should be approached cautiously.
- **Magnesium:** Supplementation may be indicated for cramps, restless legs, or laboratory-confirmed low levels. Gentle, easily

absorbed forms (magnesium citrate, glycinate) may cause fewer digestive symptoms than magnesium oxide. As excessive intake can interact with kidney function, dosing in older adults should prioritize low-to-moderate range unless otherwise directed by a physician.

- **Alpha-Lipoic Acid:** Used for diabetic or metabolic neuropathies, therapeutic doses range from 300–600mg per day in clinical trials for adults, but long-term safety in seniors is not fully established. Medication interactions (including for thyroid and diabetes drugs) are possible, so discussion with healthcare providers is crucial.
- **Omega-3 Fatty Acids:** Fish oil capsules can raise blood levels efficiently, but quality, dosage, and potential blood-thinning effects should be considered. Seniors on anticoagulant drugs or with bleeding disorders need medical oversight to avoid adverse reactions.

Basic Interactions Grid for Key Supplements:

- B12 may mask folate deficiency and interact with some anti-convulsants and metformin.
- Magnesium can interfere with absorption of certain antibiotics and osteoporosis drugs when taken simultaneously.
- High-dose B6, over time, is itself neurotoxic.
- Alpha-lipoic acid may lower blood sugar, so diabetics on medication require dose monitoring.
- Fish oil (omega-3 supplements) can enhance effects of blood thinners like warfarin or aspirin.

Rarely should supplements outright replace food sources, except in cases of absorption disorders, restrictive diets, or documented deficiencies. All changes in supplementation should be logged and communicated to healthcare teams to minimize risk of unnecessary duplication or adverse interactions.

Hydration, Digestive Health, and the Absorption Puzzle in Older Adulthood

The potential for any nutrient to improve nerve function depends not just on what is eaten, but on how well it is digested and absorbed, an aspect of special concern to older adults.

- **Hydration:** Fluids are vital for nerve signaling as well as digestion. Even mild dehydration hampers nutrient transport, slows wound healing, and exacerbates constipation problems that in turn impair the availability of B vitamins and magnesium at the cellular level. Seniors may have a weaker thirst cue and should aim for regular water intake, adjusting for personal health conditions.
- **Digestive Efficiency:** With age, stomach acid can naturally decline, medications may suppress acid further, and tooth or gum issues can limit effective chewing. These factors can undermine the release and absorption of B12, magnesium, and zinc. Slow digestion might lead to bloating or discomfort, causing reduced appetite and elimination of entire food groups. For those with frequent tummy upsets, smaller, more frequent meals and use of well-cooked or pureed options can help increase total nutrient density.
- **Absorption Barriers:** Several common medications such as proton pump inhibitors for acid reflux, metformin for diabetes,

and certain diuretics directly or indirectly reduce nutrient absorption from food. Chronic illnesses and inflammatory gut conditions intensify these effects. For seniors, even marginal deficiencies in B12 or magnesium can result in pronounced neurological symptoms.

A proactive approach includes:

- Eating a variety of textures to accommodate dental limitations.
- Favoring cooked vegetables and stews for easier chewing and absorption.
- Reviewing medications with pharmacists or doctors to monitor nutrient interference.
- Considering periodic nutrient testing, especially for B12, vitamin D, and magnesium levels in the setting of neuropathy or persistent digestive complaints.

In summary, the most sophisticated nutrition plan for nerve health is only as effective as the body's ability to process, absorb, and utilize its ingredients. Seniors benefit from a "whole system" mindset, adjusting fluid, meal timing, and supplement routines as needed to optimize internal delivery.

Building a Personalized Nutrient Base for Nerve Health

Supporting nerve function and managing neuropathy in older adulthood is less about chasing the latest superfood or supplement, and more about integrating a tailored set of nutritional building blocks with daily consistency. The synergy between balanced meals, appropriate supplementation, hydration, and digestive support yields the environment in which nerves are most likely to thrive or recover.

- Begin with the staples: Diverse, minimally processed whole foods rich in B vitamins, magnesium, omega-3s, and anti-inflammatory compounds.
- Address blood sugar and inflammation through mindful carbohydrate choices and the inclusion of healthy fats and antioxidants at every meal.
- Layer in supplements cautiously, with individual factors and medication profiles guiding safe dosing and choice.
- Monitor barriers to absorption, hydration, digestion, and medication impact keeping your care team in the loop when changes are made.

These seemingly modest actions establish the bedrock for nerve stability, comfort, and potential healing. Each nutrient, each meal, and every mindful adjustment serves as an investment not just in the relief of today's symptoms, but in the preservation of mobility, independence, and quality of life for years to come.

Anti-Inflammatory Eating for Neuropathy Management

Inflammation is a double-edged sword for seniors living with neuropathy. On one hand, the body's immune response can help repair small injuries to tissues, but when inflammation becomes chronic often fueled by dietary triggers it can silently wear down nerves over time. For older adults, where healing slows and sensitivities increase, mastering anti-inflammatory eating is not just sensible; it becomes a daily strategy for supporting comfort, function, and resilience in the face of nerve pain.

Foods work in both directions: some quiet the biological fires tied to numbness, tingling, and discomfort, while others stoke them, worsening both symptoms and underlying degeneration. Understanding these effects doesn't require advanced nutrition knowledge but it does require awareness, intention, and a willingness to experiment with what works for your own body.

Navigating the world of dietary inflammation starts with mapping which foods help protect nerves, which are safe in small amounts, and which are best left off the plate for good. Beyond simply listing foods, you'll discover how antioxidant-rich choices can help combat the "rust" of nerve cells, what a satisfying anti-inflammatory menu looks like in real life, and how to gauge your weekly habits for stealthy pro-inflammatory culprits. Let's chart a clear, sustainable course through the landscape of nutrition and nerve health.

Dietary Sources: Which Foods Help, Which Harm?

A senior's everyday meal choices introduce a wide spectrum of biochemical influences—some calming, some aggravating. While the specific impact of each food depends on one's individual biology, medications, and preferences, certain food groups are reliably associated with higher or lower levels of inflammation.

Anti-Inflammatory Foods to Prioritize:

- **Green leafy vegetables:** spinach, kale, Swiss chard, collard greens, bok choy, arugula
- **Cruciferous vegetables:** broccoli, cauliflower, Brussels sprouts, cabbage
- **Root vegetables:** carrots, beets, sweet potatoes, yams, turnips
- **Berries:** blueberries, strawberries, blackberries, raspberries
- **Fatty fish:** salmon, sardines, mackerel
- **Nuts and seeds:** walnuts, chia seeds, flaxseeds, pumpkin seeds, almonds
- **Healthy oils:** extra-virgin olive oil, avocado oil
- **Herbs and spices:** turmeric, ginger, garlic, cinnamon, rosemary, oregano, basil, mint
- **Fiber-rich fruits:** apples, pears, cherries, figs, grapes, kiwi
- **Mushrooms,** onions, leeks
- **Legumes:** lentils, beans, peas

Foods to Limit (occasional or small amounts):

- **Whole grains:** brown rice, oatmeal, barley (choose minimally processed versions)
- **Starchy vegetables:** white potatoes, corn (eat in moderation)
- **Pasture-raised eggs,** skinless poultry
- **Low-fat dairy or fortified plant milks** (if tolerated)
- **Natural sweeteners:** honey, maple syrup (use sparingly)

Foods to Avoid or Greatly Minimize:

- **Processed meats:** bacon, sausages, deli meats, hot dogs
- **Refined grains:** white bread, white pasta, pastries, crackers
- **Sugary foods:** candy, sweetened beverages, desserts
- **Fried foods:** chips, fries, doughnuts, store-bought fried snacks
- **Artificial sweeteners:** some individuals may find increased neuropathic symptoms with these
- **Excessive saturated fats:** processed snack foods, commercial baked goods, many fast foods
- **Alcohol:** significant intake may worsen nerve irritation
- **Foods with high sodium:** canned soups, frozen meals, heavily salted snacks

This approach is not about strict denial, but about tilting everyday food choices toward options that feed resilience rather than irritation. Meals built heavily from the "prioritize" column give the body daily supplies of the nutrients and phytochemicals most protective for nerves and circulatory health.

Antioxidants and Polyphenols: Shielding Nerves from Oxidative Stress

Oxidative stress is a silent process where free radicals and unstable oxygen molecules damage the integrity of nerve cells, much like how metal rusts or apples brown when cut open. For seniors, particularly those with diabetes, post-shingles pain, or age-related metabolic decline, this stress accelerates nerve dysfunction and the sensations of burning, numbness, or stabbing pain.

Antioxidants are molecules that serve as molecular guardians, neutralizing free radicals and reducing their destructive potential. Polyphenols, a special group of antioxidants found in plant foods, go a step further: they can block inflammatory signals and support healthy blood vessel function, keeping oxygen and nutrients flowing to vulnerable nerves.

Protective Antioxidant and Polyphenol Sources:

- **Berries:** rich in anthocyanins and vitamin C
- **Dark leafy greens:** abundant in carotenoids, vitamin E, folate
- **Spices:** turmeric (curcumin), cinnamon, ginger—potent anti-inflammatory agents
- **Colorful vegetables:** carrots, bell peppers, squash, tomatoes
- **Olive oil:** polyphenols support microcirculation and cell defense
- **Green tea:** catechins stabilize cellular defenses
- **Nuts and seeds:** vitamin E, selenium
- **Beans and lentils:** polyphenols, fiber, magnesium

Eating a rainbow of colors is more than aesthetic; it maximizes the diversity of antioxidants and polyphenols, ensuring overlapping layers of defense for nerve cells. Aim to include at least one or two rich sources at each meal. This habit can meaningfully lower the burden of oxidative stress that accelerates nerve degeneration.

A Sample Day: Anti-Inflammatory Meal Plan in Practice

Applying anti-inflammatory nutrition is simpler when you can visualize how a day's eating might look, balancing flavor, color, variety, and practicality for seniors.

Breakfast: Berry-Chia Oat Bowl

- Rolled oats slow-cooked with unsweetened almond milk, topped with fresh blueberries, a sprinkle of chia seeds, diced walnuts, and ground cinnamon
- 1 cup green or mint tea

Mid-Morning Snack: Sliced pear with a small handful of almonds

Lunch: Lentil-Spinach Soup with Avocado Toast

- Vegetable broth simmered with cooked lentils, chopped spinach, carrots, celery, seasoned with turmeric and garlic
- 1 slice whole-grain toast, spread with mashed avocado, sprinkled with flaxseed

Afternoon Snack: Sliced cucumber and carrot sticks with hummus dip

Dinner: Baked Salmon with Roasted Vegetables

- Salmon fillet brushed with olive oil, lemon, and fresh dill, baked until tender
- Roasted Brussels sprouts, sweet potato wedges, and red bell peppers
- Quinoa salad with parsley, cherry tomatoes, and lemon vinaigrette

Evening "Golden Milk": Steamed oat milk blended with turmeric, black pepper, and a pinch of ginger

This menu provides anti-inflammatory, antioxidant-rich ingredients in every meal and snack. Portions can be adapted for appetite, swallowing ability, or satiety. Ingredients like lentils, salmon, berries, nuts, and greens target multiple nutrition needs at once, offering steady fuel, blood sugar balance, and cell repair support for seniors.

The Inflammation Scorecard: Reflecting on Weekly Choices

It's easy to lose track of patterns across a week; one indulgent meal blends into the next, and the sum effect may creep past your intended boundaries. For anyone aiming to reduce nerve pain by lowering inflammation, a simple self-rating tool can help you stay on course.

This Inflammation Scorecard is not about guilt; it's a reflective tool to help you spot trends that could be influencing symptoms and to gently nudge habits in a better direction.

Rate the following for each day of the week, then add up your weekly total.

For Each Day, Score as Follows:

3 points: Ate mostly from anti-inflammatory foods (lots of vegetables, berries, healthy fats, lean proteins, herbs, and spices; few processed or sugary foods)2 points: Balanced; mostly whole foods, but one or two servings of refined grains, processed snacks, or sweets1 point: Frequent processed foods, sugars, refined grains, or fried items; few vegetables or anti-inflammatory foods

Weekly Score (Out of 21 possible points):

18–21: Excellent. Consistent anti-inflammatory eating. Your nerves and blood vessels likely feel the benefit.14–17: Good. Some days drifted, but the overall pattern supports nerve health. Fine-tune for even better stability.10–13: Fair. Inflammatory foods are slipping in more often than not.

Consider meal prepping, shopping adjustments, or new recipes.Below 10: Potential trigger for inflammatory symptoms. Consider a focused reset return to the food lists, seek support, and discuss with a care team if symptoms worsen or don't improve.

This self-assessment helps translate daily choices into a broader view reminding you that each week is a new opportunity to shift the balance toward healing foods.

Spotting and Reducing Dietary Triggers in Everyday Life

Many seniors recognize certain symptoms spike after shared meals, holidays, or convenience foods, but pinpointing the culprits can be tricky. Several categories of food are well-documented for their ability to enhance chronic inflammation, make blood sugar swings more pronounced, and, over time, worsen neuropathy symptoms.

Common Dietary Triggers to Watch:

1. **Processed and Deli Meats:** These foods are high in preservatives, sodium, and unhealthy fats. Not only can they directly promote inflammation, but regular consumption may also contribute to circulatory issues, putting nerves at further risk.
2. **Refined Grains:** Foods like white bread, pasta, crackers, and pastries are stripped of their fiber and nutrients. They turn quickly to sugar in the bloodstream, triggering blood sugar surges that hasten nerve injury—especially problematic in diabetes.
3. **Added and Excess Sugars:** Sweetened drinks, desserts, candies, and even "hidden sugars" in sauces accelerate inflammation and oxidative stress. They also undermine the stability of blood sugar, which is central to nerve health management in seniors.
4. **Unhealthy Fats and Fried Foods:** Commercial deep-fried snacks, chips, and processed baked goods offer unhealthy fats that actively feed inflammation and oxidative nervous system injury. Fast foods, with their combination of salt, fat, and sugar, pose a particular risk for both microcirculation and nerve tissue.
5. **Artificial Sweeteners and Alcohol:** Some individuals report greater sensitivity and increased neuropathic symptoms with

regular use of aspartame, sucralose, or excessive alcohol intake. Where possible, choose natural sweeteners sparingly if needed, and limit or avoid alcohol to protect nerve stability.

The intent is not to ban favorite foods forever but to recognize their position on the inflammation spectrum. Occasional small servings of a favorite meal are unlikely to undo a week of anti-inflammatory eating, but regular, daily exposure to these triggers can quietly shift your baseline toward discomfort and slower recovery.

How to Minimize Inflammatory Triggers

Start with Awareness: Keep a simple food-mood-symptom log for a week. Note energy, sensation changes, pain spikes, and foods eaten at meals or snacks.

1. **Swap and Substitute:** Replace white bread with whole-grain, swap fries for roasted sweet potato wedges, and season meals with fresh herbs and spices instead of salty sauces.
2. **Batch Prep Anti-Inflammatory Meals:** Prepare simple vegetable-forward soups, stews, or grain salads in advance, making healthy choices more convenient.
3. **Request Modifications:** When eating with family or at group meals, ask for sauces or dressings on the side, or bring a favorite healthy dish to share.
4. **Shop the Perimeter:** In grocery stores, spend most of your trip in the produce, fish, and bulk grain sections, avoiding packaged snacks and sweets.

Support Systems for Success

Reducing inflammation through food requires more than an understanding of lists. Setting up your home environment and routines makes healthy default choices easier and reduces the daily energy spent on decisions.

- Keep washed and cut vegetables available for grab-and-go snacks.
- Store fresh and frozen berries, leafy greens, and herbs within eyesight in the fridge or freezer.
- Invest in small containers for nuts, seeds, and trail mixes for portable, nutrient-rich snacks.
- Rotate through different herbs and spices to keep meals flavorful and interesting—palate fatigue can reduce enjoyment over time, especially with age-related taste shifts.
- If swallowing, chewing, or appetite problems arise, consult with your doctor or a registered dietitian for tailored solutions. Sometimes pureed soups, stews, or smoothies can deliver the same benefits in an accessible form.

When to Seek Additional Advice

While anti-inflammatory nutrition is powerful, some contributors to inflammation such as medication side effects or underlying health changes are outside the scope of food. If you experience unexplained increases in nerve pain, new areas of numbness, rapid loss of sensation, or marked difficulty with daily eating, reach out to your healthcare provider promptly. Periodic check-ins ensure your nutrition plan flexes alongside changes in medications, health status, or life circumstances, and a registered dietitian can help refine your eating patterns for maximum nerve support.

Mastering anti-inflammatory eating for neuropathy is a dynamic, lifelong process. It is guided by broad scientific principles, refined by individual response, and empowered by the knowledge that small changes, repeated daily, deliver real benefits for comfort and function.

By integrating a variety of colorful, whole-food ingredients into your meals, focusing on herbs, healthy fats, and reducing inflammation triggers, you gradually shift your body's terrain from one of vulnerability to one of resilience. A tracking habit whether with a scorecard, a weekly meal plan, or a symptom journal helps maintain both awareness and control, making progress visible and rewarding.

With each thoughtful grocery trip, every vibrant plate, and every check-in with your support team, you carve a path toward steadier nerve health and the quality of life you deserve. The following chapters will guide you through practical strategies for achieving these aims, even when physical or energy barriers stand in the way laying out recipes, tactics, and everyday solutions so the science of anti-inflammatory nutrition becomes your lived reality.

Senior-Specific Kitchen and Meal Planning Tools

"Why does cooking suddenly feel so much harder than it used to?" That question, quietly voiced by countless older adults, gets to the heart of managing neuropathy in the kitchen. Numbness, pain, and reduced hand strength make the once-simple tasks of meal prep chopping, stirring, lifting pots newly complicated. Fluctuating appetite, dry mouth, diminished taste, or blurry vision further reshape the eating experience. With a few vital adjustments, both kitchen routines and meal planning can serve the needs of nerve health without exhausting energy or confidence.

Unlike standard meal guides, this chapter recognizes and addresses the lived realities of seniors with neuropathy: hands that fumble, eyes that strain, shoulders that tire quickly, and appetites that fluctuate. The following strategies, tools, and ready-to-use planning aids translate the science of anti-inflammatory eating into daily routines that are safe, satisfying, and sustainable.

Adapting the Kitchen: Practical Setups for Mobility, Dexterity, and Vision

Traditional kitchens may feel like obstacle courses to those living with neuropathy. Reduced grip strength, joint stiffness, and altered sensation in the hands call for layouts and tools tailored for safety and ease.

Choosing the right location for meal prep makes a difference. Whenever possible, arrange the workspace so all essentials, chopping boards, knives, bowls are within easy reach to reduce unnecessary walking or reaching. Lightweight and anti-slip mats minimize risks of utensils or bowls sliding off the counter. Pull-out shelves or baskets at waist level eliminate the need for frequent bending or stretching.

Investing in a few senior-friendly kitchen tools can relieve joint pain and reduce accidents. Ergonomic utensils, such as knives with easy-grip handles and spring-loaded scissors, minimize strain and help maintain control while cutting or peeling. Adaptive jar openers and electric can openers spare tender fingers and wrists. Consider color-contrasting cutting boards and utensils for those with reduced vision, making ingredient preparation easier to track visually.

For stovetop safety, opt for heavier pans that won't tip easily, but only if their weight is manageable. Cookware with two handles distributes weight for safer lifting. Induction burners provide immediate-on, immediate-off heating for seniors who may become distracted, as they cool rapidly if left unattended.

Lighting matters: ample overhead and focused task lighting reduces mistakes and strain. In kitchens where space is tight or clutter accumulates, a rolling cart loaded with meal prep essentials can turn any area into an accessible workspace.

Preparing ingredients in advance such as peeling and chopping vegetables or portioning proteins—is wise, especially during times of higher energy or less pain. Freezing or refrigerating these foods in clear, labeled containers allows for quick, low-effort assembly later, removing the pressure to cook from scratch for every meal.

Portion Management, Safe Food Handling, and Sensory Support

For seniors, a safe kitchen is not just about avoiding burns or cuts; it's about matching portion sizes to appetite, navigating meal prep with diminished sensation, and defending against foodborne illness—something those with slower healing must take seriously.

Start with portion control. Standard serving spoons and scoops may be hard to maneuver; instead, pre-portion staple foods like cooked whole grains, vegetable sides, or proteins into small, sealable containers for the week ahead. Using color-coded measuring cups or divided plates makes it easier to maintain visual consistency in meal sizes, simplifying nutrition tracking and preventing accidental over- or under-eating.

Safe food handling means prioritizing food that's easy to chew and swallow, prepared with utmost attention to doneness and hygiene. Always check perishable foods for changes in smell, color, or texture before eating. For those with numb fingers, investing in vegetable scrubbers, cut-resistant gloves, and automatic soap dispensers adds a protective layer when washing and prepping ingredients.

Meal prepping with sensory changes in mind calls for variety in color, aroma, and texture, which stimulate appetite even when taste or smell is dulled. Combining hot and cold elements, arranging foods with vibrant vegetables or colorful fruits, and seasoning with fresh herbs and citrus can liven up both the plate and the palate. Small containers of pre-chopped veggies, sliced fruit, or classic dips (like hummus or guacamole) reduce on-the-spot prep and make nutrient-rich snacking convenient. When possible, choose produce already washed and cut, or ask for help assembling ingredients for major meal batches.

Traditional knives and graters may be hard to grip if sensation is reduced. Food processors, mandolines with safety guards, or simply opting for pre-cut produce can ease effort; they remove fine motor demands while preserving nutritional quality. Large, easy-to-read kitchen timers minimize the risk of burning food or forgetting a step, allowing for distraction or a rest mid-prep.

Aids like microwave or oven-safe plates and bowls, fitted with handles or insulation, aid in lifting without a firm grip. Silicone baking mats or parchment paper minimize the mess and cleanup burden, important for those with reduced energy or hand mobility. Lastly, avoid stacking or piling dishes dangerously high; drying racks that catch drips and keep plates upright remove the need to towel-dry each piece individually.

Visual Meal Planning: Mapping a Week for Energy and Nutrients

Planning a week's meals does more than cut down time in the kitchen; it's a way of making anti-inflammatory nutrition habitual, visually ensuring balance across food groups and nutrients. For seniors managing neuropathy, a visual meal planner is especially helpful for memory, organization, and energy conservation.

A calendar grid with spaces labeled for breakfast, lunch, dinner, and snacks for each day of the week. On this planner, place concise cues:

- Color-code meals by protein source (e.g., blue for fish, green for plant proteins, red for poultry).
- Icons or stickers to indicate days with new recipes, batch-prepared leftovers, or a "slow-cooker" night.
- Highlighted boxes to mark at least one serving of leafy greens and colorful vegetables at lunch and dinner.
- Circles or checkmarks to show inclusion of a healthy fat source such as olive oil, avocado, or nuts at each meal.

This planner can be posted on a fridge, pinned near the pantry, or kept on a tablet for accessible viewing. The visual format ensures several things: that high-fiber, nutrient-rich foods anchor the week; protein and healthy fat intake stays consistent; and processed food options do not dominate out of convenience fatigue.

A sample visual planner for seniors might look like this for a typical midweek:

Monday:

- **Breakfast:** Veggie omelet, whole grain toast, orange slices
- **Snack:** Green smoothie (spinach, mango, banana, almond milk)
- **Lunch:** Hummus and vegetable sandwich, lentil soup
- **Snack:** Chopped carrots/cucumber and hummus
- **Dinner:** Baked salmon with broccoli and sweet potato

Tuesday:

- **Breakfast:** Peanut butter banana oat shake
- **Snack:** Raspberries and almond butter
- **Lunch:** Grilled eggplant and tomato pasta salad
- **Snack:** Handful of walnuts, dried apricots
- **Dinner:** Rosemary chicken with spinach and beans, balsamic salad

Customize these maps based on food preferences, energy levels, and any scheduled outings or social meals. Keeping portable snacks noted on busier days guards against skipped meals, which can lower blood sugar and worsen neuropathy symptoms.

Affordable, Longevity-Focused Shopping List Templates

Grocery shopping is a skill and an act of self-care for those living with nerve pain. Leaning into food choices that last, fit a realistic budget, and fill the anti-inflammatory pantry pays dividends when energy or appetite fluctuates.

The following template puts anti-inflammatory foods front and center, grouped for easy reference and smart purchasing.

Proteins:

- Eggs
- Salmon, cod, or other oily fish (fresh, frozen, or canned)
- Chicken breast, turkey
- Beans, lentils, chickpeas (canned or dried)
- Tofu, hummus
- Greek yogurt (plain) or unsweetened plant-based yogurt

Produce (fresh and frozen for flexibility):

- Spinach, kale, Swiss chard
- Broccoli, Brussels sprouts, carrots, beets
- Sweet potatoes, winter squash
- Berries (fresh or frozen strawberries, raspberries, blueberries)
- Apples, pears, oranges

Pantry and Healthy Fats:

- Olive oil, avocado oil
- Walnuts, almonds, pumpkin seeds, sunflower seeds
- Flaxseed, chia seeds
- Quinoa, brown rice, whole grain pasta
- Spices: turmeric, ginger, cinnamon, garlic, rosemary, basil

Shelf-stable and Bulk:

- Rolled oats
- Low-sodium vegetable stock
- Tomato paste, stewed tomatoes
- Nut butters (unsweetened)

This template can be used on paper, laminated for repeated use, or filled digitally for online ordering. Prioritize items with longer shelf life like dried beans, frozen vegetables, or canned fish during times of reduced mobility or when shopping trips must be less frequent.

For extra savings, opt for store brands, shop sales for bulk nuts and seeds, and substitute with whatever fresh produce is in season. Do not overlook frozen or bagged produce; they are picked at peak ripeness, nutritionally robust, and reduce waste if eating happens in smaller portions.

Pay attention to ingredient lists: avoid foods with added sugars, excess sodium, or chemical preservatives. Focus instead on the shortest lists, with ingredients you recognize as whole foods. For those who do not use a full container quickly, storage in small, clear containers improves both visibility and durability.

Overcoming Appetite Loss, Chewing Troubles, and Taste Changes

Many seniors with neuropathy face a dwindling desire to eat, dry mouth, oral health challenges, and taste changes that make previously-loved meals seem bland or unappealing. Good nutrition remains critical for nerve protection and general resilience so adapting the eating experience is non-negotiable.

To encourage appetite and consistent eating, rely on smaller, more frequent meals. Lightly schedule snacks between main meals to avoid long stretches without intake. If breakfast or dinner feels overwhelming, halve typical portions and enjoy nutrient-dense snacks throughout the day: sliced fruit with nut butter, Greek yogurt with berries, or a small smoothie that blends greens with banana for a gentle, easy-to-swallow option.

Texture and temperature adaptation matters for those with chewing or swallowing problems. Offer softer foods, soups, stews, vegetable purees, smoothies, and slow-cooked grains. Whole grains like oatmeal or quinoa can be cooked extra-soft and mixed with pureed fruit, diced eggs, or soft cheese for variety and fullness. Use sauces, gravies, or broths to moisten dry foods and ease swallowing.

Seasoning plays a role in revitalizing the palate. When taste or smell diminishes, experiment with lemon juice, vinegar, fresh herbs, ginger, or citrus zest instead of salty sauces or heavy dressings. Rotate flavors and textures alternate a tangy green salad with a creamy vegetable soup, or follow a crunchy snack with a soft fruit compote. Chilled foods, such as fruit smoothies or yogurt parfaits, may be especially helpful for those with oral discomfort or burning mouth sensations.

Dental issues can further hinder chewing. Choose ground meats, flaky baked fish, or emulsified spreads (hummus, guacamole) for ease. Canned or stewed fruits and vegetables can be just as nutritious and require less work to eat. If dentures or missing teeth are an issue, cut foods into bite-sized pieces, and avoid hard-crusted breads or raw, tough vegetables.

For dry mouth, keep a glass of water or herbal tea at hand, or try sugarless lozenges to promote saliva. Avoid caffeine-heavy or salted snacks, which can worsen dehydration.

For significant or ongoing difficulties with appetite, chewing, or swallowing, a consultation with your healthcare provider or a registered dietitian is essential. Dental care and medication review may uncover reversible causes, and individualized nutrition counseling can further adapt your plan.

By adapting the kitchen environment, using accessible and safe equipment, batch-prepping meals, and maintaining visual structure through planners and lists, the daily work of eating for nerve health becomes more manageable even as body and sensory changes present new puzzles to solve. The central aim is not just to "get by," but to maintain autonomy, pleasure, and steady nerve support, all while defending against malnutrition and meal fatigue.

Living with neuropathy may set limits, but smart tools and strategies let you reclaim control over what you eat and how you prepare it. A thoughtfully arranged kitchen, infused with low-effort, high-nutrient options, can be a senior's best buffer against both nerve flares and meal-time frustration.

As you move forward in this guide, take time to try the templates, experiment with new tools, and ask for help where needed. With practice, the science-backed principles of anti-inflammatory eating can be lived day-to-day: not just in recipes, but in every choice that makes the kitchen safer, the meal more nourishing, and the process more joyful.

28-Day Neuropathy Recovery Plan: Week-by-Week System

The start of any recovery process is rarely linear, and even the most thoughtfully designed meal or lifestyle plan is not simply a checklist to be ticked once and forgotten. Instead, meaningful change happens through structure, incremental progress, and gentle self-awareness. The following 28-day system maps out a stepwise path to help seniors living with neuropathy, whatever the underlying cause, stabilize daily habits, reduce symptom burdens, and regain a feeling of control around eating, movement, and self-care. Unlike generic meal challenges or one-size-fits-all nutrition plans, this approach is grounded in the distinct needs and experiences of older adults, paying attention to the realities of nerve pain, energy swings, and unpredictable appetite.

The plan unfolds in four clearly marked phases, each with its focus and realistic milestones. This chapter walks you through the system week-by-week, layering habits, behavioral observations, and troubleshooting advice so the process remains as adaptable as it is ambitious. Along the way, you'll find prompts for self-assessment, moments to reorient after setbacks, and a set of behavioral cues to notice so you can respond to your body's signals with compassion not judgment.

Charting the 28 Days: Phased Progress, Not Perfection

The structure of the 28-day neuropathy recovery plan is engineered to support gradual adoption and steady self-discovery rather than racing to an endpoint. Each phase builds upon the previous one, allowing new routines the space to become familiar before advancing to the next layer of complexity.

Phase 1: Stabilize (Days 1–7)

- Core Focus: Begin consistent meal timing, boost hydration, and eliminate high-glycemic and highly processed foods.
- Expected Progress: Initial reduction in symptom spikes tied to erratic blood sugar or dehydration; gentler digestive responses; fewer drastic appetite swings.

Phase 2: Nourish (Days 8–14)

- Core Focus: Incorporate targeted anti-inflammatory foods at each meal. This includes at least two servings of colorful vegetables per day and the use of olive oil or avocado oil with at least one meal.
- Expected Progress: Notable improvements in bowel regularity, modest decrease in daily pain or numbness intensity, more stable energy—especially in the afternoon.

Phase 3: Activate (Days 15–21)

- Core Focus: Layer in gentle, senior-appropriate movement (e.g., short chair-based exercises), and increase protein quality (fish, beans, eggs) to further support nerve health. Continue strict avoidance of processed snacks and excess sugars.

- Expected Progress: Improved mobility, less morning stiffness, smaller windows of daily fatigue. Gradual sense of regained strength or resilience.

Phase 4: Empower (Days 22–28)

- Core Focus: Enhance mind-body connection through daily self-tracking, stress management tactics (like deep breathing at meals), and refining meal prep routines for independence.
- Expected Progress: Greater confidence in adapting meals or snacks to daily needs. Sharper awareness of what triggers or relieves symptoms. Possible improvements in both mood and balance, though progress may remain variable.

Each phase is not just about adding new tasks. Instead, old habits are reviewed and adjusted as needed. For some seniors, progress may seem slow, or particular steps (e.g., increasing raw vegetable intake or new exercise routines) may take extra time. What matters is continued engagement not rigid adherence to a calendar.

Building Core Habits, One Day at a Time

Most nutrition plans focus on what to eat, but experience shows it's the scaffolding of daily habits when you eat, hydrate, move, and reflect that underpins real change for older adults. The following timeline serves as both a habit blueprint and a gentle contract with yourself over the course of the month.

Week 1:

- Wake with a glass of water before breakfast. Hydration first, even before coffee or tea.
- Schedule three meals at regular intervals (e.g., 8 am, 12:30 pm, 6 pm), with optional snacks based on hunger.
- Track meals and symptoms (pain, tingling, mood) at the end of each day using a simple paper or digital log.
- Begin or continue a minimum of 5 minutes of mindful movement daily: stretching, range-of-motion seated moves, or gentle walks with support as needed.

Week 2:

- Increase non-caffeinated fluid intake to at least six cups per day if medically appropriate. Add a second glass of water with each meal.
- Introduce a wide variety of colorful vegetables (fresh, frozen, or lightly cooked) at both lunch and dinner.
- Maintain regular mealtimes; reduce meal skipping even on low appetite days by shifting to smaller or softer items rather than nothing at all.
- Continue daily movement, expanding by 2-3 minutes if comfortable, and record energy levels during or after activity.

Week 3:

- Evaluate if two fish-based meals or vegetarian protein options (like lentils or beans) are included per week. If not, add them to the menu or swap in nutrient-rich equivalents.
- Try a new form of gentle physical activity if ready (e.g., guided chair yoga or resistance bands), adjusting for safety.

- Consolidate hydration by positioning water bottles or cups in high-visibility areas (bedside, living room, kitchen).
- Evaluate consistency in meal logging and movement; address gaps by setting reminders or enlisting support.

Week 4:

- Set aside a specific time daily perhaps after breakfast or before dinner to fill out a short self-assessment (see tool at the chapter's end).
- Revisit pantry and fridge for processed packaged foods; swap lingering high-sodium items, sweets, or snack bars for fiber-rich or whole food alternatives.
- Practice a brief daily stress-relief method: slow breathing, gratitude journaling, or savoring food scents before eating.
- Tally up the previous week's symptom trends and note progress, setbacks, or plateaus.

By laying out a visible, day-by-day plan, you anchor the larger commitment of nerve health into specific, manageable actions. Whether you use check marks on a calendar, dots on a tracking form, or short notes in a symptom log, the act of daily recordkeeping is critical not just for accountability but for building a feedback loop between lifestyle and change.

Tuning In: Recognizing Behavioral Cues

Older adults with neuropathy often live with dull or distorted signals from nerves, muscles, and even the digestive system. Focusing attention on behavioral cues helps build intuition for what your body now needs, versus old habits or routine.

Anticipate these cues as signs to pause and respond with appropriate self-care:

- **Hunger:** For some, neuropathy blunts appetite, but classic cues may still appear—stomach growling, irritability, fatigue, or lightheadedness. If you no longer notice these, schedule small meals at regular intervals.
- **Thirst:** Dry mouth, thick saliva, headache, or even confusion may appear before a true feeling of thirst, as a sense of fluid need may fade with age or nerve changes. If you wake with a parched feeling or struggle to swallow dry foods, increase non-caffeinated liquids.
- **Fullness:** Numbness, abdominal bloating, or a prolonged sense of heaviness after eating may indicate fullness before classic satiety cues are triggered. Slow your eating, pause between bites, and stop when even slight discomfort appears.
- **Blood sugar shifts:** Sudden fatigue, shakiness, vision changes, or headaches can mean blood sugar is dropping or spiking. Eating balanced, measured meals with fiber and healthy fats helps, but keep a high-fiber snack or small protein option at hand for unexpected lows.
- **Symptom flare-ups:** A burning or tingling intensity, a sense of "electricity" in the feet or hands, swelling, or muscle cramps often signal that something—meal timing, food choice, hydration, or even stress requires adjustment.

By paying close attention to these signals and adapting the day's plan as needed, you reinforce mindfulness while decreasing the risk of overcorrection (like overeating or chronic underhydration).

Course-Correcting: What to Do When Setbacks Strike

Missed meals, days of low energy, or a sudden return of symptoms are not reasons to abandon the plan, but inherent parts of living with nerve changes. The most effective recovery approaches are those that embrace setbacks as learning opportunities, not failures.

If you miss a meal:

- Don't try to "make up" for it by doubling the next plate. Instead, eat a regular-sized meal at your next scheduled time, and keep a portable snack of nut butter on whole grain bread, Greek yogurt with fruit, or a banana at the ready for true hunger pangs later in the day.

On days of low energy:

- Prioritize hydration. Fatigue often comes from mild dehydration or undernutrition. Sip on water or herbal tea, and opt for easy-to-assemble foods: a veggie omelet, a simple smoothie, or canned beans on whole grain toast.
- Limit physical demands, but maintain some movement to encourage circulation—standing stretches, arm raises while seated, or a slow walk to the mailbox.

When symptoms flare:

- Review your meal and hydration log. Were high-sugar or processed foods eaten more than usual? Was a meal or snack skipped? Sometimes, even small lapses can trigger symptoms.

- If symptoms persist or worsen rapidly, consult your healthcare provider, as medication adjustments or clinical evaluation may be needed.

If tracking falls behind or feels overwhelming:

- Shrink the task. Instead of writing detailed notes, use a simple system: smiley or frown faces to mark days with fewer or more symptoms, or colored dots to indicate pain intensity. Enlist a friend or caregiver if digital tools are easier than pen and paper.

Addressing setbacks in this compassionate, flexible manner keeps the process from becoming punitive. The goal is resilience, not rigid compliance.

Weekly Self-Assessment Worksheet: Bridging Awareness and Action

At the end of each week, a regular self-check provides a snapshot of your progress, highlights subtle improvements, and flags areas that need more focus. Use the following worksheet adapted or simplified to personal comfort to reflect on where you stand and what adjustments might support the coming week.

28-Day Neuropathy Recovery Plan: Weekly Self-Assessment

Circle or mark your answers for each question. Review your responses with your healthcare provider or use them to adjust your next week's plan.

1. **How would you describe your average pain level this week?**

- No pain
- Mild discomfort
- Moderate, managed with rest or food
- Severe, affecting daily activity

2. **Rate the frequency of numbness or tingling in hands or feet.**

- Never
- 1-2 days
- 3-5 days
- Daily

3. **How was your energy for daily tasks?**

- Very good; did most things I wanted
- Good, with some limits
- Low; struggled with common routines
- Very low; unable to do most things

4. **Did you notice any changes in mood (e.g., improved outlook, more frustration, more hope, less interest)?**

- Improved
- Mostly steady
- Up and down
- More negative than before

5. What changes did you make to meals, movement, or hydration this week? (Open space for notes)
6. List any foods, drinks, or activities that seemed to worsen or help your symptoms. (Open space for notes)
7. Did you need help with meals, movement, or tracking? If yes, what kind and by whom?

8. Are there new questions or worries to discuss with your medical provider or caregiver?

The reason this system succeeds is not just its nutritional bases, but in how it transforms daily actions. A regular routine of meal timing, hydration, and gentle movement supports blood sugar stability, decreases inflammation, and helps prevent the spikes and dips that worsen neuropathy. Core foods, especially vegetables; protein-rich options, including eggs, fish, and legumes; olive oil or other healthy fats; and whole, fiber-rich grains form the foundation. Just as essential is the commitment to regular self-review and nonjudgmental course corrections.

Progress rarely looks like a straight climb; instead, it cycles, plateaus, and sometimes regresses. The genuine transformation comes with consistency: marking your daily choices, responding to behavioral cues, and approaching setbacks as part of your unique path forward.

In the chapters ahead, you will find the practical tools to further personalize your neuropathy-supportive diet, anti-inflammatory recipes, stepwise meal preparation, and adaptable strategies. This phased, week-by-week plan gives you a flexible yet evidence-backed roadmap.

Whether you're just beginning to reshape your habits or have years of experience managing neuropathy, ongoing structure and compassionate self-awareness will help you keep building a life where meals, movement, and daily choices support not just your nerves, but your sense of independence and hope.

Nerve-Supporting Recipes, Part 1—Breakfasts, Snacks, and Smoothies

Breakfast, snack, and smoothie recipes for seniors with neuropathy ought to do more than merely fill a plate they need to deliver targeted nutrients in ways that are easy to prepare, enjoyable to eat, and mindful of inflamed nerves, changes in appetite, and physical challenges that often come with age. For this first recipe collection, the journey starts not with rules, but with real meals: 20 options that blend anti-inflammatory foods, classic comfort, and practical kitchen wisdom.

Each recipe is detailed to help you shop, prep, and serve, even if grip, vision, or energy sometimes fall short. Along the way, you'll find ways to batch-cook, freeze, adjust for allergies, and substitute ingredients to keep nerve health a top priority at every meal.

Why Breakfasts, Snacks, and Smoothies Matter

When nerve pain or numbness complicates eating, skipping early meals or grazing on processed carbs can lead to unpredictable blood sugar, spikes in discomfort, and mood swings. By contrast, mindful choices, especially those rich in B vitamins, magnesium, antioxidants, healthy fats, and lean white proteins set the foundation for steadier energy and fewer symptom flares during the day.

The recipes that follow reflect this approach, harnessing foods like leafy greens, omega-3-rich seeds, berries, and eggs to help decrease inflammation and support nerve signaling from the start of your day.

Twenty Senior-Friendly Recipes: Breakfasts, Snacks, and Smoothies

Every recipe includes a senior-friendly prep note with tips for easier handling, batch-prep options, and the most useful substitutions. For those living alone or cooking with fatigue, several dishes are designed for 1–2 servings, with batch-cooking adaptations for convenience.

Spinach-Olive Oil Frittata

Ingredients:

- 2 large eggs
- 1 cup fresh spinach, roughly chopped
- 1 small onion, diced
- 1 tablespoon olive oil
- Pinch of sea salt and black pepper

Instructions:

1. Heat olive oil in a nonstick skillet over medium. Add the onion; cook, stirring, 4 minutes.
2. Add spinach and cook until wilted, about 1 minute.
3. Beat eggs with salt and pepper; pour over vegetables.
4. Cover and cook 5–7 minutes until set; use a spatula to loosen edges and slide onto a plate.

Senior prep note: Pre-chopped spinach and pre-diced onions save energy.

Berry-Chia Yogurt Parfait

Ingredients:

- 1 cup plain Greek yogurt (or unsweetened plant yogurt)
- ½ cup mixed berries (blueberries, raspberries, strawberries)
- 1 tablespoon chia seeds
- 1 tablespoon chopped walnuts

Instructions:

1. In a glass or bowl, layer yogurt, berries, chia seeds, and walnuts.
2. For a softer texture, let sit 10 minutes before eating.

Prep note: Use frozen berries if fresh are costly or unavailable.

Turmeric-Apple Smoothie

Ingredients:

- 1 apple, cored and chopped
- ½ cup unsweetened almond or oat milk
- 1 teaspoon ground turmeric
- 1 tablespoon almond butter
- ½ teaspoon cinnamon
- ½ frozen banana

Instructions:

1. Add all ingredients to a blender; process until creamy.
2. Add extra milk to thin if needed.

Prep note: Slicing and freezing bananas ahead saves effort and provides extra creaminess.

Green Smoothie

Ingredients:

- 2 cups spinach
- 2 cups water
- 1 cup mango
- 1 cup pineapple
- 2 bananas (at least one should be frozen for chill)

Instructions:

1. Pack spinach into a blender with water; blend until smooth.
2. Add mango, pineapple, and bananas; blend again until silky.

Prep note: Use mixed frozen fruits for simplicity; works well as batch-prepped freezer packs.

Quick Oatmeal with Pumpkin Seeds and Blueberries

Ingredients:

- ½ cup rolled oats
- 1 cup water or milk of choice
- 2 tablespoons pumpkin seeds
- ½ cup blueberries

Instructions:

1. Combine oats and liquid in a small pot; bring to a simmer.
2. Cook 5 minutes until thick; stir in pumpkin seeds and blueberries.

Prep note: Make several servings at once, refrigerate, and reheat as needed.

Peanut Butter Banana Oat Shake

Ingredients:

- ¼ cup rolled oats
- ¼ cup water
- 1 cup milk of choice
- 1 large ripe banana
- 1–2 tablespoons unsweetened peanut or almond butter
- 2 teaspoons honey (or to taste)
- ¼–½ teaspoon ground nutmeg
- 2 ice cubes (optional)

Instructions:

1. Combine oats and water in a microwave-safe bowl; microwave 1 minute, cool.
2. In a blender, add cooked oats, milk, banana, nut butter, honey, nutmeg, and optional ice. Blend until smooth.

Prep note: Pre-cook oats in batches, portion, and freeze to stir into quick shakes.

Savory Sweet Potato Toast

Ingredients:

- 1 medium sweet potato
- 1 tablespoon olive oil
- ½ avocado, mashed
- Salt, pepper, and pinch of smoked paprika

Instructions:

1. Slice sweet potato lengthwise into ¼-inch slabs.
2. Brush with oil; bake at 400°F for 20 minutes or until soft.
3. Cool, top with avocado, season, and eat warm or cold.

Batch tip: Make a tray of sweet potato "toast" for several days' snacks.

Cottage Cheese, Berry, and Walnut Bowl

Ingredients:

- ¾ cup cottage cheese (dairy or non-dairy)
- ½ cup berries
- 2 tablespoons chopped walnuts
- 1 teaspoon honey (optional)

Instructions:

1. Scoop cottage cheese into a bowl.
2. Top with berries, walnuts, and drizzle with honey if desired.

Prep note: For soft foods, mash berries before adding.

Veggie Omelette

Ingredients:

- 2 large eggs
- ¼ red pepper, chopped
- ¼ cup cheddar cheese, grated
- Small handful spinach leaves
- 2 cherry tomatoes, chopped
- Salt and pepper
- ¼ teaspoon butter

Instructions:

1. Cut tomatoes, peppers, and spinach.
2. Whisk eggs, season, and pour into a heated pan with butter.
3. Top with veggies and cheese; cook over medium until set, fold, and serve.

Prep note: Use pre-chopped or frozen vegetables.

Hummus and Vegetable Snack Plate

Ingredients:

- ½ cup hummus
- 1 cup mixed raw veggies: carrots, cucumber slices, bell pepper strips
- 1 hard-boiled egg (optional)

Instructions:

1. Arrange veggies and eggs on a small plate.
2. Serve with hummus for dipping.

Batch tip: Pre-slice veggies and keep in airtight containers for easy reach.

Berry-Almond Energy Bites

Ingredients:

- 1 cup rolled oats
- ½ cup almond butter
- ¼ cup honey
- ¼ cup dried cranberries or cherries
- ¼ cup chopped almonds
- 1 tablespoon chia seeds

Instructions:

1. Mix all ingredients in a bowl; roll into 1-inch balls.
2. Refrigerate 1 hour to firm up.

Prep note: Make double batches, freeze extras for future snacking.

Chia Pudding with Mango

Ingredients:

- 4 tablespoons chia seeds
- 1 cup unsweetened coconut milk
- ½ cup diced mango

Instructions:

1. Stir chia and coconut milk in a bowl; let rest 15 minutes, stirring once.
2. Top with mango and serve.

Batch tip: Make several portions at once; refrigerate up to 4 days.

Apple-Cinnamon Quinoa Breakfast Bowl

Ingredients:

- ½ cup cooked quinoa
- ½ apple, diced
- 2 tablespoons raisins
- 1 teaspoon cinnamon
- 2 teaspoons chopped walnuts
- ½ cup milk of choice

Instructions:

1. Warm quinoa with milk in a saucepan.
2. Stir in apple, raisins, and cinnamon. Serve topped with walnuts.

Prep note: Use leftover quinoa for efficiency.

Avocado-Berry Smoothie

Ingredients:

- 1 ripe avocado
- 1 cup unsweetened almond milk
- ½ cup berries
- 1 tablespoon sunflower seeds
- 1 teaspoon lime juice

Instructions:

1. Add all ingredients to the blender; blitz until creamy.

Prep note: Halve avocado and freeze directly in the peel for ready access.

Greek Yogurt and Peach Bowl

Ingredients:

- 1 cup plain Greek yogurt
- 1 diced ripe peach or ½ cup thawed frozen peaches
- 1 tablespoon flaxseed

Instructions:

1. Combine all ingredients in a bowl.
2. Stir and enjoy.

Substitution: Use canned fruit in juice, drained, if fresh is unavailable.

Walnut-Blueberry Snack Squares

Ingredients:

- 1 cup quick oats
- ½ cup mashed banana
- ½ cup chopped walnuts
- ¼ cup dried blueberries or cranberries
- 2 tablespoons olive oil

Instructions:

1. Mix all ingredients; press into a parchment-lined loaf pan.
2. Bake at 350°F for 15 minutes. Cool and cut into squares.

Batch tip: Wrap and freeze individually for quick snacks.

Grilled Eggplant Salad (Snack/Lunch)

Ingredients:

- 1 eggplant, sliced into rounds
- 2 tablespoons olive oil
- 1 red bell pepper, chopped
- ½ red onion, sliced
- 1 tablespoon chopped parsley

Instructions:

1. Brush eggplant with oil, grill or broil until soft.
2. Toss with peppers, onion, and parsley. Drizzle with a bit more olive oil.

Prep note: Use pre-grilled or jarred eggplant strips for speed.

Roasted Chickpeas

Ingredients:

- 1 can (15 oz) chickpeas, drained and rinsed
- 1 tablespoon olive oil
- ½ teaspoon smoked paprika
- ¼ teaspoon turmeric

Instructions:

1. Pat chickpeas dry; toss with oil and spices.
2. Spread on a baking sheet; roast at 400°F for 25 minutes, shaking halfway.

Batch tip: Cool completely; store in an airtight container for crunchy snacks for up to a week.

Almond Butter and Pear Toast

Ingredients:

- 1 slice whole-grain bread
- 1 tablespoon almond butter
- ½ ripe pear, thinly sliced
- Dash cinnamon

Instructions:

1. Toast bread, spread with almond butter, layer pear slices, dust with cinnamon.

Substitution: *Use seed butter for nut allergies.*

Veggie & Hummus Sandwich

Ingredients:

- 2 slices whole grain bread or a gluten-free wrap
- ¼ cup hummus
- ½ cup shredded carrot
- ¼ cup sliced cucumber
- 2 tablespoons alfalfa sprouts or leafy greens

Instructions:

1. Spread hummus on bread; top with veggies and greens, assemble.

Portion note: Halve for a small snack or serve whole for a meal.

Table: Which Nerve-Support Nutrients Are in Each Recipe?

To simplify ingredient choices and help you match recipes to your specific needs, this table maps each recipe to its most prominent nerve-support nutrients.

Recipe	B12	Omega-3s	Antioxidants	Magnesium/Other
Spinach-Olive Oil Frittata	eggs	—	spinach, onion	spinach
Berry-Chia Yogurt Parfait	yogurt	chia seeds, walnuts	berries	chia, walnuts
Turmeric-Apple Smoothie	—	almond butter	apple, turmeric	almond butter
Green Smoothie	—	—	spinach, pineapple, mango	spinach, banana
Oatmeal with Seeds	—	pumpkin seeds	blueberries	oats, pumpkin seeds
Peanut Butter Banana Shake	—	peanut butter	banana	oats, peanut butter
Sweet Potato Toast	—	—	sweet potato, avocado	sweet potato
Cottage Cheese, Berry & Walnut	cottage cheese	walnuts	berries	walnuts
Veggie Omelette	eggs, cheese	—	spinach, tomatoes, peppers	—

Hummus & Veggies Plate	egg (if added)	—	carrots, peppers	hummus
Berry-Almond Energy Bites	—	almond butter, chia	dried fruit	almonds, chia
Chia Pudding w/Mango	—	chia seeds	mango	chia
Apple-Cinnamon Quinoa Bowl	—	walnuts, flax	apple, raisins	walnuts, quinoa
Avocado-Berry Smoothie	—	sunflower seeds	berries	avocado, seeds
Greek Yogurt & Peach Bowl	yogurt	flaxseed	peaches	flax
Walnut-Blueberry Squares	—	walnuts	blueberries, cranberries	walnuts
Grilled Eggplant Salad	—	olive oil	eggplant, pepper, parsley	eggplant
Roasted Chickpeas	—	—	turmeric	chickpeas
Almond Butter/Pear Toast	—	almond butter	pear, cinnamon	almond
Veggie & Hummus Sandwich	—	—	carrot, cucumber	hummus

Tactics for Batch-Prepping, Freezing, and Rotating Meals

Batch preparation can be a game changer for those with unpredictable energy or mobility. Several strategies reduce day-to-day effort and ensure that anti-inflammatory, nerve-supportive choices are always at hand:

- Double or triple recipes like oatmeal, chia pudding, and energy bites, then portion into single servings for the fridge or freezer. Use freezer-safe containers with easy-open lids for arthritis-friendly access.
- For frittatas, omelettes, and baked breakfast squares, cook in a large pan, then cool and cut into wedges or squares. Store in individual containers safe to refrigerate for up to 4 days or freeze for up to 2 months. Reheat gently in the microwave or toaster oven.
- Smoothie packs simplify daily blending. Pre-portion all solid smoothie ingredients (except liquids) into zip-top bags and freeze. In the morning, just add liquid, blend, and serve.
- Roasted vegetables and chickpeas last for several days refrigerated. Use top salads, combine with grains, or add to wraps through the week.
- Label all freezable items clearly with recipe name and date. Rotate older items to the front of your fridge or freezer for first use, minimizing spoilage and stress.
- Snack plates and cut veggies can be prepped on a weekend day, stored in small containers, and grabbed for hunger between meals.

Portion Guides and Substitutions for Common Allergens or Dietary Restrictions

Seniors often need tailored portions and ingredient swaps based on personal needs or doctor recommendations. **Here are adaptable guidelines:**

Portioning:

- **Breakfasts:** Aim for protein-rich options (one frittata wedge, ¾–1 cup of yogurt bowl, ½ cup of cooked grains, or 2 eggs/omelets).
- **Snacks:** Stick with a piece of fruit, a handful (1–2 ounces) of nuts/seeds, ½–¾ cup of smoothie, or a small bowl of energy bites (2–3).
- **Smoothies:** Typically 8–10 ounces per serving for most seniors. Easy to divide or adjust according to hunger and medication timing.

Those with dental concerns may blend solid snacks or use softer cooked versions.

Substitution Strategies:

- **Dairy-free:** Replace cow's milk or yogurt with unsweetened almond, oat, or coconut versions. Choose fortified varieties when possible to supply vitamin B12 and calcium.
- **Egg-free:** Substitute chickpea flour "scrambles" or tofu for frittatas and omelettes.

- **Nut allergies:** Use sunflower or pumpkin seed butter in place of almond or peanut butter. Choose seeds instead of nuts as toppings.
- **Gluten-free:** Opt for certified gluten-free oats and breads, or serve breakfast bowls in leafy greens instead.
- **Lower sodium:** Use fresh herbs and spices in place of added salt. Rely on naturally flavorful ingredients (citrus, vinegar, garlic, fresh herbs) to compensate.
- **Sugar restriction:** Skip honey or use unsweetened applesauce or pureed fruit to sweeten. Allow the natural sweetness of fruit to shine, especially in smoothies and puddings.
- **Vegetarian or vegan:** Most recipes are inherently plant-focused; for extra protein, choose soy yogurt, plant-based milks, or tofu scrambles.

Recipe Spotlight: Walking Through an Example

Take the Spinach-Olive Oil Frittata, a recipe simple enough for beginners yet layered with ingredients proven to support nerve and overall health. Spinach delivers fiber, magnesium, and protective phytonutrients; eggs supply high-quality protein and B12; olive oil brings anti-inflammatory fats. Seniors can whisk eggs in a bowl, use a pre-chopped vegetable medley, and let the stovetop do most of the work. If gripping a pan is difficult, a silicone spatula makes for easy lifting.

For those who like to plan ahead, double the recipe and store extra portions in the refrigerator for up to four days. Pair with a side of fresh berries for an added antioxidant boost.

Making Healthy Eating Routine—With Confidence

Eating well with neuropathy doesn't have to mean complicated cooking or bland meals. By focusing on anti-inflammatory ingredients, senior-friendly preparation techniques, and flexible batch-cooking strategies, these recipes make it easier to nourish your nerves and enjoy food every day. Remember to adjust portions and ingredients as needed for your preferences and any dietary restrictions.

With this collection of 20 breakfasts, snacks, and smoothies, you're equipped to make mornings brighter, snacks more satisfying, and each meal a step toward better nerve health.

Nerve-Supporting Recipes, Part 2—Soups, Salads, and Light Lunches

Lunchtime holds a special place in the daily rhythm of older adults managing neuropathy. After the reliable comfort of breakfast, midday meals are a chance to bring in a second wave of nerve-friendly nutrients, sustained energy, and flavor diversity without weighing down the digestive system or sapping stamina with complicated prep.

For those living with neuropathic pain, tremor, or numbness, ease matters as much as nutrition. The following 20 soups, salads, and light lunches draw on a pantry of anti-inflammatory ingredients, streamlined assembly, and modifications that make mealtime safer and more enjoyable for those with sensory changes.

Convenience does not have to mean compromise. Many of the dishes below can be made in advance, adapted for small-batch or family-style eating, and modified for individual needs. Each recipe features detailed ingredient quantities, methods adjusted for people with limited dexterity or grip strength, and tips for adapting heat levels to both flavor and nerve comfort. The result is a toolkit of meal options that reward the effort, support nerve function, and make lunch one of the most inviting and least stressful moments of the day.

20 Senior-Optimized Recipes: Soups, Salads, Light Lunches

Roasted Carrot-Lentil Soup

Ingredients:

- 1 pound carrots, peeled and sliced
- 1 cup cooked lentils (canned or pre-steamed)
- 1 medium yellow onion, chopped
- 2 cloves garlic, peeled
- 3 cups low-sodium vegetable broth
- 2 tablespoons olive oil
- ½ teaspoon ground cumin
- ½ teaspoon ground turmeric
- ¼ teaspoon black pepper
- Optional: juice of ½ lemon, chopped fresh parsley

Instructions:

1. Preheat the oven to 400°F. Spread carrots, onion, and garlic on a baking tray; drizzle with olive oil and roast for 25 minutes until soft.
2. Tip roasted vegetables into a pot with lentils, broth, cumin, turmeric, and pepper.
3. Simmer for 10–15 minutes. Use an immersion blender or potato masher for your preferred consistency.
4. Stir in lemon juice and parsley before serving.

Accessibility tip: Use pre-peeled carrots and pre-chopped onion to reduce prep steps.

Quinoa-Avocado Salad

Ingredients:

- 1 cup cooked quinoa (warm or cold)
- 1 ripe avocado, diced
- ½ cup cherry tomatoes, halved
- ¼ cup cucumber, diced
- 2 tablespoons pumpkin seeds
- 2 tablespoons chopped fresh basil or parsley
- 1 tablespoon lemon juice or apple cider vinegar
- 1 tablespoon olive oil
- Pinch sea salt and pepper

Instructions:

1. In a large bowl, gently combine all ingredients, folding in avocado last.
2. Drizzle with lemon juice and olive oil; toss until just combined.

Stepwise assembly: Buy pre-cooked quinoa or steam a batch in advance. Use a fork to mash avocado if dicing is difficult.

Herb Chicken Lettuce Wraps

Ingredients:

- 1 pound ground chicken breast
- 1 cup diced jicama
- 1 cup cooked brown rice
- 1 cup halved and thinly sliced English cucumber
- ½ cup fresh cilantro leaves
- 16 Bibb or butter lettuce leaves
- 4 tablespoons creamy peanut butter
- 2 tablespoons low-sodium soy sauce
- 2 tablespoons honey
- 2 tablespoons water
- 2 teaspoons toasted sesame oil
- 2 teaspoons olive oil
- 3 scallions, sliced
- 1 tablespoon minced fresh ginger
- 2 teaspoons minced fresh garlic
- 1 serrano pepper, seeded and minced (optional)
- Lime wedges for serving

Instructions:

1. For sauce, whisk peanut butter, soy sauce, honey, water, sesame oil, olive oil, white parts of scallion, ginger, garlic, and pepper in a bowl.
2. In a nonstick skillet, cook ground chicken until browned. Mix in jicama and half the sauce, heat until just warmed.

3. Place cooked rice, chicken mixture, cucumber, and cilantro in lettuce leaves. Serve with lime wedges and remaining sauce for drizzling.

Technique note: Pre-chopped veggies speed assembly; lettuce leaves can be gently separated with hands instead of knives.

Grilled Eggplant Salad

Ingredients:

- 1 medium eggplant, cut into ½-inch slices
- 1 medium red bell pepper, stemmed, seeded, and quartered
- ½ medium red onion, peeled and cut into 1-inch wedges
- 1 cup halved cherry tomatoes
- ¾ cup chopped flat-leaf parsley
- ¼ cup sliced scallions
- ¼ cup chopped fresh mint
- 1 teaspoon lemon zest
- 3 tablespoons lemon juice (divided)
- ¼ cup olive oil
- ½ teaspoon salt
- 2 teaspoons za'atar or Italian seasoning
- Cooking spray

Instructions:

1. Preheat grill or broiler to medium-high; coat vegetables with oil and za'atar.
2. Grill vegetables until soft and browned (about 5–7 minutes per side).
3. Cool veggies, then dice or slice as able. Mix with tomatoes, parsley, scallions, mint, lemon, and salt. Toss well.
4. Serve at room temperature or slightly chilled.

Motor adaptation: Use jarred, pre-grilled eggplant and chopped bell peppers in place of grilling.

Chickpea-Spinach Soup

Ingredients:

- 1 can (15 oz) chickpeas, rinsed and drained
- 4 cups low-sodium vegetable broth
- 2 cups baby spinach (or frozen spinach)
- 1 medium carrot, diced (use pre-diced if preferred)
- 1 small onion, chopped
- 2 cloves garlic, minced
- 1 teaspoon cumin
- 1 tablespoon olive oil
- Pepper to taste

Instructions:

1. Heat olive oil in a pot. Add onions, carrot, and garlic; cook until softened.
2. Add chickpeas, broth, cumin, and pepper. Simmer for 20 minutes.
3. Stir in spinach. Cook 2–3 more minutes until wilted.

Cooling note: Let soup cool before serving to avoid burns for those with reduced tactile sensation.

Salmon and Green Bean Niçoise Salad

Ingredients:

- 1 cooked salmon fillet (baked or poached)
- 2 cups mixed salad greens
- ½ cup cooked green beans, cut into 2-inch pieces
- 1 small potato, steamed and diced
- 2 hard-boiled eggs, sliced
- ¼ cup black olives
- 2 tablespoons Olive oil
- 1 tablespoon lemon juice
- 1 tablespoon chopped parsley

Instructions:

1. Arrange greens, green beans, potatoes, eggs, and olives on a plate. Flake salmon and place on top.
2. Drizzle with olive oil and lemon juice; sprinkle with parsley.

Assembly short-cut: Use canned salmon and pre-cooked green beans and potatoes for minimal prep.

Lentil, Beet, and Walnut Salad

Ingredients:

- 1 cup cooked lentils (pre-steamed)
- 1 medium cooked beet, diced (store-bought or microwaved)
- 2 cups mixed leafy greens
- ¼ cup walnuts, chopped
- ¼ cup diced cucumber
- 2 tablespoons balsamic vinegar
- 1 tablespoon olive oil
- ¼ teaspoon salt

Instructions:

1. Toss lentils, beet, greens, walnuts, and cucumber in a bowl.
2. Drizzle with vinegar and oil; toss very gently.

Accessibility: Consider steamed lentils and pre-cooked beets, available in many produce sections.

Sweet Potato-Black Bean Burgers (as a lunch patty)

Ingredients:

- 2 cups grated sweet potato
- 1 cup no-salt-added black beans, rinsed
- ½ cup oats, ground
- ½ cup chopped scallions
- ¼ cup vegan mayonnaise or Greek yogurt
- 1 tablespoon tomato paste
- 1 teaspoon curry powder
- ⅛ teaspoon salt
- 4 whole-wheat burger buns (optional)

Instructions:

1. Squeeze water from sweet potato; combine with all ingredients in a bowl.
2. Mash together and form into patties.
3. Cook in a skillet over medium heat, turning once, until crispy on both sides.
4. Serve warm, with or without buns, over greens or cucumbers.

Finger strength tip: Mash mixture with hands for more control if mixing with a spoon is difficult.

Balsamic-Spinach Berry Salad

Ingredients:

- 2 cups baby spinach leaves
- ¼ cup mixed berries (blueberries, blackberries, or strawberries)
- ¼ cup crumbled feta or goat cheese
- ¼ cup toasted walnuts or pecans
- 2 tablespoons balsamic vinaigrette (see below)

Vinaigrette:

- 2 tablespoons aged balsamic vinegar
- 2 tablespoons Dijon mustard
- 1 tablespoon maple syrup or honey
- ¼ teaspoon kosher salt
- 6 tablespoons olive oil

Instructions:

1. Whisk vinaigrette ingredients in a jar.
2. Lightly toss salad ingredients with dressing.

For limited grip: Use bagged baby spinach and ready-washed berries; crumble cheese directly into salad.

Steamed Veggie Bowl with Turmeric Rice

Ingredients:

- 1 cup steamed brown rice (microwavable or leftover)
- ½ cup steamed broccoli florets
- ½ cup steamed cauliflower
- ½ zucchini, sliced and steamed
- 1 tablespoon olive oil
- ½ teaspoon turmeric
- Pinch black pepper
- 1 tablespoon sunflower or pumpkin seeds

Instructions:

1. Combine rice with turmeric and pepper; toss to color grains evenly.
2. Pile veggies on top. Drizzle with olive oil, sprinkle seeds for crunch.

Assembly: Opt for pre-cut vegetable steamer bags from the produce section.

Cucumber-Dill Yogurt Soup (cold)

Ingredients:

- 1 large cucumber, peeled and diced
- 1 cup plain Greek yogurt
- 2 tablespoons chopped fresh dill
- 1 small clove garlic, grated
- 2 teaspoons lemon juice
- Pinch sea salt

Instructions:

1. Blend all ingredients in a blender until smooth.
2. Chill at least 1 hour; serve cold with a drizzle of olive oil and extra dill.

For those with sensitive teeth: Let soup sit at room temperature briefly before eating.

Broccoli-Almond Soup

Ingredients:

- 2 cups broccoli florets (fresh or frozen)
- 1 cup low-sodium vegetable broth
- 2 tablespoons almond butter
- 1 tablespoon olive oil
- Pinch of nutmeg
- Salt and pepper, to taste

Instructions:

1. In a saucepan, simmer broccoli in broth until soft.

2. Add almond butter; blend until creamy with an immersion blender.
3. Stir in olive oil, nutmeg, salt, and pepper.

Motor note: Use a microwaveable steamer bag for broccoli to minimize cutting.

Chickpea-Herb Salad Pita

Ingredients:

- 1 cup canned chickpeas, rinsed and smashed lightly with fork
- 2 tablespoons olive oil
- 2 tablespoons chopped parsley
- 1 scallion, thinly sliced
- ½ teaspoon lemon zest
- 1 tablespoon lemon juice
- Pinch black pepper
- 2 small whole-wheat pitas

Instructions:

1. Mix all salad ingredients; stuff evenly into pitas.

Assembly: Fork-mashing the chickpeas is easier than using a food processor.

Spiced Pumpkin Soup

Ingredients:

- 1 can (15 oz) pumpkin purée
- 2 cups low-sodium chicken or vegetable broth
- ½ onion, finely diced
- 1 teaspoon grated ginger
- ½ teaspoon ground cumin
- ½ teaspoon cinnamon
- 1 tablespoon olive oil
- Salt and pepper

Instructions:

1. Sauté onion in olive oil until translucent, add ginger and spices.
2. Stir in pumpkin and broth, simmer for 10–15 minutes.
3. Blend for smoothness if desired.

Heating safety: Let soup cool to below steaming before ladling into bowls.

Spring Pea and Mint Salad

Ingredients:

- 2 cups spring mix greens
- ½ cup thawed frozen green peas
- 2 tablespoons chopped fresh mint
- 1 tablespoon lemon juice
- 1 tablespoon olive oil
- 2 tablespoons crumbled feta

Instructions:

1. Toss greens, peas, and mint lightly.
2. Dress with lemon juice, olive oil, and sprinkle with feta.

Grip tip: Use a salad spinner with a push-down handle if rinsing greens at home.

Avocado-Tomato Bulgur Bowl

Ingredients:

- 1 cup cooked bulgur wheat
- 1 ripe avocado, diced
- ½ cup cherry tomatoes, halved
- 2 tablespoons chopped scallions
- 1 tablespoon lemon juice
- 1 tablespoon olive oil
- Salt and pepper

Instructions:

1. Mix bulgur, avocado, tomatoes, and scallions.
2. Dress with lemon juice, olive oil, and toss gently.

Carbohydrate note: Bulgur is high in fiber and easy to chew; substitute quinoa for gluten-free diets.

Red Lentil Vegetable Stew

Ingredients:

- 1 cup red lentils, rinsed
- ½ cup chopped carrots
- 1 cup chopped celery
- 1 small tomato, diced
- 1 small onion, chopped
- 4 cups water or vegetable broth
- 1 tablespoon olive oil
- ½ teaspoon ground cumin

Instructions:

1. Bring all ingredients to a boil in a pot, reduce to simmer; cook for 20 minutes until lentils are tender.

<u>Kale-Pear-Walnut Salad</u>

Ingredients:

- 2 cups chopped kale (remove stems)
- ½ ripe pear, sliced
- ¼ cup walnuts
- 1 tablespoon lemon juice
- 1 tablespoon olive oil
- 1 tablespoon raisins (optional)

Instructions:

1. Massage kale leaves with lemon juice and oil to soften.
2. Add pear, walnuts, and raisins; toss well.

Adaptation: Pre-chopped bagged kale saves time and reduces cutting.

Cauliflower-Apple Soup

Ingredients:

- 2 cups cauliflower florets
- 1 apple (peeled, chopped)
- 2 cups low-sodium vegetable broth
- ½ small onion, chopped
- 1 tablespoon olive oil
- ½ teaspoon dried thyme

Instructions:

1. Sauté onion in olive oil; add cauliflower, apple, broth, and thyme.
2. Simmer until soft, blend for creamy consistency.

Reheating note: Microwave portions in short increments, stirring between to prevent scalding.

Hummus & Veggie Wrap

Ingredients:

- 1 large whole-wheat or gluten-free wrap
- ¼ cup hummus
- ½ cup shredded carrot
- ½ cup baby spinach
- ¼ cup shredded red cabbage
- ¼ cup sliced cucumber

Instructions:

1. Spread hummus over wrap; layer veggies evenly.
2. Roll and slice into bite-size pieces for easier handling.

Prep tip: Pre-shredded veggies reduce risk of knife slips and simplify assembly.

Ingredient Sourcing for Value and Ease

Smart shopping is as important to nerve health as smart cooking, especially for seniors on fixed incomes or with limited mobility. **Choose stores that offer these time- and budget-saving options:**

- Buy pre-washed greens, pre-chopped vegetables, and steam-in-bag produce.
- Utilize canned beans and lentils (low sodium, rinsed) for salads and soups.
- Look for pre-cooked whole grains like quinoa, brown rice, and bulgur in the deli or freezer section.
- Choose shelf-stable cartons of low-sodium broth for soups.
- Favor frozen fruits and vegetables when fresh is not available or affordable—they are just as nutritious and last longer.
- Purchase nuts and seeds in bulk; portion into small containers to preserve freshness.

Whenever possible, plan meals around weekly store specials, in-season produce, and pantry staples such as olive oil, vinegar, dried herbs, and legumes. These ingredients not only stretch the food budget, but help ensure a constant supply of nerve-supportive nutrients.

Accessible Assembly: Stepwise Meal Preparation

Many older adults with neuropathy experience finger numbness, pain, or limited grip strength. Adapting meals for varying abilities makes cooking both safer and more enjoyable.

For most recipes, start with these step-by-step principles:

1. Assemble all ingredients on the counter before beginning plastic bowls with grippy bottoms to prevent sliding.
2. Use pre-chopped, pre-washed, or frozen vegetables to reduce the need for peeling and dicing.
3. For mixing, choose large-handled utensils or silicone spatulas; heavy glass bowls may offer more stability than lightweight plastic.
4. Use jarred minced garlic and ginger rather than mincing by hand.
5. When opening jars, opt for a rubber grip pad or an electric jar opener to minimize strain on the hands. If using cans, select those with easy-pull tabs, or invest in an ergonomic can opener designed for limited dexterity.
6. Consider prepping ingredients in seated positions at a table with non-slip mats to steady bowls and boards. Slow down and take breaks as needed to avoid fatigue. Cooking is not a race, and pacing helps prevent accidents.
7. If cutting is required, use a sharp, lightweight knife and a cutting board with a damp towel underneath for extra stability. For especially tough jobs, such as slicing dense vegetables, ask a family member or caregiver for help, or choose pre-cut options whenever possible.
8. Keep frequently used tools like measuring cups, spatulas, and towels within easy reach to avoid unnecessary bending or stretching. Small changes in set-up and technique can make a

big difference, transforming lunchtime prep from a source of frustration into an empowering daily ritual.

By combining thoughtful ingredient choices with accessible cooking strategies, older adults managing neuropathy can enjoy nourishing, delicious lunches that honor both taste and ability.

Nerve-Supporting Recipes, Part 3—Hearty Dinners and Comfort Meals

For many older adults living with neuropathy, dinnertime is more than a final meal—it is comfort after a long day and an occasion to restore both body and spirit. Hearty main dishes and satisfying sides become anchors for stable blood sugar, improved satiety, and a signal to wind down. Unlike lighter soups or salads, dinner invites richer flavors, more substantial proteins, and the warmth of cooked comfort. The potential challenges of meal preparation reduced grip strength, impaired sensation, changing tastes mean these recipes must deliver both practical ease and nourishment.

What follows is a carefully curated series of 25 anti-inflammatory dinners and sides, each tailored for fullness, senior accessibility, nerve health, and the pleasure of eating well. From slow-cooker stews to colorful roasted vegetables, these dishes combine tried-and-true kitchen science with sensory adaptations, so that any older adult managing neuropathy can navigate the evening meal with satisfaction and confidence.

Anti-Inflammatory, Senior-Friendly Main Dishes and Sides

Each dinner recipe included here has been selected for its balance of fiber, complex carbohydrates, healthy fats, and lean protein. Most also feature vibrant vegetables rich in antioxidant and anti-inflammatory compounds berries, dark leafy greens, orange squashes, beans, and seeds have all shown promising effects in lowering chronic inflammation and supporting nerve health.

Within these recipes, you'll see substitutions for common allergens, diabetes-friendly modifications, and techniques for those requiring softer textures or simplified assembly. The sequence of meals below covers a variety of world cuisines, classic comfort fare, and approachable senior staples:

Baked Salmon with Walnut-Crust and Roasted Veggies

Ingredients:

- 4 salmon fillets (about 3 ounces each)
- ⅓ cup walnuts, finely chopped
- 1 tablespoon Dijon mustard
- 1 tablespoon honey or sugar-free substitute
- 2 teaspoons olive oil
- 1 teaspoon low-sodium tamari or soy sauce
- Fresh ground black pepper
- 1 medium red bell pepper, cut into ½-inch pieces
- 1 small eggplant, cut into ½-inch pieces
- 1 medium yellow squash, cut into ½-inch pieces
- 1½ cups butternut squash, peeled and cubed

Instructions:

1. Preheat the oven to 425°F. Line a baking sheet with parchment paper.
2. Toss all vegetables in olive oil, pepper, and a splash of balsamic vinegar. Spread on the baking sheet and roast for 10 minutes.
3. Mix mustard, honey, and tamari. Brush salmon lightly with the mixture. Sprinkle chopped walnuts onto each fillet; press gently to help them adhere.
4. Add salmon fillets atop the vegetables. Roast for another 12 minutes, until fish flakes easily and veggies are soft.

Sweet Potato Mash

Ingredients:

- 2 large sweet potatoes, peeled and cubed
- 2 tablespoons plain Greek yogurt or vegan yogurt
- 1 tablespoon olive oil
- ¼ teaspoon ground cinnamon (optional)
- Pinch sea salt

Instructions:

1. Boil sweet potato cubes in salted water for 15 minutes or until very soft.
2. Drain and mash while still hot, adding yogurt, olive oil, and cinnamon.
3. Serve warm for a soothing, blood-sugar-friendly side.

Lentil Shepherd's Pie

Ingredients:

- 1½ cups cooked brown or green lentils
- 2 carrots, diced
- 1 cup frozen peas
- 1 medium yellow onion, chopped
- 1 cup low-sodium vegetable broth
- 2 tablespoons olive oil
- 2 teaspoons dried thyme
- 2 cups Sweet Potato Mash (see above)

Instructions:

1. Preheat the oven to 375°F. Sauté onion and carrot in oil until soft.
2. Stir in lentils, broth, peas, and thyme. Simmer for 10 minutes until the mixture thickens.
3. Spoon into a baking dish; top evenly with mashed sweet potatoes.
4. Bake for 20 minutes until the topping is lightly browned.

Garlic-Tahini Steamed Greens

Ingredients:

- 1 bunch Swiss chard or kale, ribs removed and leaves chopped
- 2 tablespoons tahini
- 2 tablespoons lemon juice
- 1 clove garlic, minced
- 1 tablespoon olive oil
- 2 tablespoons warm water
- Pinch salt

Instructions:

1. Steam greens in a covered pot with a splash of water until wilted (5–7 minutes).
2. Whisk together tahini, lemon juice, garlic, olive oil, and water until smooth.
3. Drizzle over warm greens before serving.

Classic Rosemary Chicken with Spinach and Beans

Ingredients:

- 4 boneless, skinless chicken breasts
- 2 teaspoons dried rosemary
- ½ teaspoon sea salt or substitute
- ½ teaspoon black pepper
- 4 teaspoons olive oil
- 6 ounces baby spinach
- 2 garlic cloves, minced
- 1 can (15 ounces) cannellini beans, rinsed and drained
- 1 can (14.5 ounces) stewed tomatoes, drained and chopped (reserve juice)

Instructions:

1. Pound chicken to ¼-inch thickness. Rub each piece with rosemary, salt, and pepper.
2. Heat half the oil in a large skillet over medium heat. Cook chicken 5–6 minutes per side; remove and keep warm.
3. In the same skillet, sauté garlic in remaining oil, add spinach until wilted, then stir in beans, tomatoes, and a splash of reserved juice. Warm through, serve with chicken.

Quinoa-Stuffed Bell Peppers

Ingredients:

- 4 large bell peppers, halved and seeded
- 1 cup cooked quinoa
- ½ cup canned black beans, rinsed
- ½ cup corn (frozen or fresh)
- 1 cup diced tomatoes
- 1 teaspoon cumin
- 1 teaspoon smoked paprika
- 2 tablespoons chopped cilantro

Instructions:

1. Preheat the oven to 375°F. Mix quinoa, beans, corn, tomatoes, cumin, and paprika.
2. Fill pepper halves with mixture. Place in a baking dish, cover with foil, and bake for 25 minutes. Uncover, top with cilantro, and bake for 5 more minutes.

Miso-Tahini Glazed Cod

Ingredients:

- 4 cod fillets
- 2 tablespoons white miso
- 2 tablespoons tahini
- 1 tablespoon lemon juice
- 1 teaspoon honey
- 1 tablespoon olive oil

Instructions:

1. Mix miso, tahini, lemon juice, honey, and olive oil. Brush onto cod fillets.
2. Bake at 400°F for 10–12 minutes, until the fish is opaque and flakes easily.

One-Pan Roasted Chicken and Autumn Vegetables

Ingredients:

- 1½ pounds chicken thighs
- ½ sweet potato, peeled and diced
- 1 carrot, sliced
- ½ lb brussels sprouts, halved
- 1 head broccoli, florets cut thick
- 2 tablespoons olive oil
- 2 tablespoons fresh rosemary, chopped
- 2 tablespoons fresh thyme, chopped
- 4 garlic cloves, minced
- Salt and pepper

Instructions:

1. Preheat the oven to 425°F. Arrange veggies and chicken on a parchment-lined sheet.
2. Toss with oil, rosemary, thyme, garlic, salt, and pepper.
3. Bake for about 30 minutes or until vegetables are fork-tender and chicken is cooked through.

Sweet Potato-Black Bean Burgers

Ingredients:

- 2 cups grated sweet potato
- ½ cup rolled oats, ground
- 1 cup no-salt-added black beans, rinsed
- ½ cup chopped scallions
- ¼ cup vegan mayonnaise
- 1 tablespoon tomato paste
- 1 teaspoon curry powder
- ⅛ teaspoon salt

Instructions:

1. Squeeze extra moisture from sweet potato. Combine everything in a large bowl and mash together.
2. Shape into patties, chill for 30 minutes.
3. Heat olive oil in a skillet, cook patties 3 minutes on each side. Serve on toasted whole-grain buns, with side salad.

Lemon-Dill Baked Trout

Ingredients:

- 4 trout fillets
- 2 tablespoons lemon juice
- 2 tablespoons chopped fresh dill
- 1 tablespoon olive oil
- ½ teaspoon sea salt

Instructions:

1. Preheat the oven to 400°F. Place trout on a parchment-lined baking sheet.
2. Drizzle with lemon, dill, oil, and salt.
3. Bake for 12–14 minutes until opaque.

Polenta with Mushroom Ragu

Ingredients:

- 1 cup quick-cooking polenta
- 2½ cups low-sodium vegetable broth
- 2 tablespoons olive oil
- 2 cups sliced mushrooms
- 1 small onion, chopped
- 2 cloves garlic, minced
- 1 tablespoon tomato paste
- 1 teaspoon dried oregano

Instructions:

1. Prepare polenta in broth per package instructions.
2. In a skillet, sauté onion, mushrooms, and garlic in olive oil. Add tomato paste, oregano, cook until thickened.
3. Spoon ragu over warm polenta.

Broccoli and White Bean Bake

Ingredients:

- 2 cups broccoli florets
- 1 can cannellini beans, rinsed
- 1 cup cherry tomatoes, halved
- 2 tablespoons chopped fresh basil
- 2 tablespoons olive oil
- 1 tablespoon lemon juice
- ¼ cup grated Parmesan or vegan cheese

Instructions:

1. Preheat the oven to 375°F. Mix all ingredients in a baking dish.
2. Roast 25 minutes until bubbling and lightly browned.

Ginger-Garlic Shrimp Stir-Fry

Ingredients:

- 1 pound raw shrimp, peeled and deveined
- 2 cups sugar snap peas or broccoli
- 1 red bell pepper, sliced
- 1 tablespoon ginger, grated
- 2 cloves garlic, minced
- 1 tablespoon coconut oil
- 1 tablespoon low-sodium tamari

Instructions:

1. Heat coconut oil in wok or skillet. Add ginger and garlic, sauté 1 minute.
2. Add shrimp and veggies; stir-fry until shrimp is pink and vegetables are crisp-tender.
3. Splash with tamari before serving.

<u>Spiced Vegetable and Chickpea Tagine</u>

Ingredients:

- 1 can chickpeas, rinsed and drained
- 2 cups butternut squash, cubed
- 1 small sweet potato, cubed
- 1 large carrot, sliced
- 1 onion, chopped
- 2 cups low-sodium vegetable broth
- 1 teaspoon ground cumin
- 1 teaspoon ground ginger
- 1 teaspoon cinnamon
- 2 tablespoons olive oil

Instructions:

1. In a heavy pot, heat oil; sauté onion. Add remaining vegetables and spices, stir to coat.
2. Add broth and chickpeas, bring to boil, then simmer 30 minutes until vegetables are tender.

Balsamic Glazed Chicken Breasts

Ingredients:

- 4 boneless, skinless chicken breasts
- 2 tablespoons balsamic vinegar
- 1 tablespoon honey
- 1 tablespoon olive oil
- 1 teaspoon dried basil

Instructions:

1. Whisk vinegar, honey, oil, and basil. Brush on chicken.
2. Bake at 375°F for 25 minutes, basting halfway.

Sautéed Spinach and Cannellini Beans

Ingredients:

- 2 tablespoons olive oil
- 2 cloves garlic, minced
- 6 ounces baby spinach
- 1 can (15 ounces) cannellini beans, rinsed and drained
- Pinch sea salt and black pepper

Instructions:

1. Heat oil in a skillet, add garlic until fragrant.
2. Add spinach, stir to wilt. Stir in beans, salt, and pepper, cook until just heated through.

Creamy Avocado and Lemon Pasta

Ingredients:

- 12 ounces gluten-free or whole grain pasta
- 1 ripe avocado
- 3 tablespoons olive oil
- 2 tablespoons lemon juice
- 2 tablespoons chopped fresh basil
- Pinch of black pepper

Instructions:

1. Cook pasta, reserving ½ cup cooking water.
2. In a blender, process avocado, olive oil, lemon juice, basil, and pepper until smooth.
3. Toss with pasta and a bit of cooking water if needed.

Oven-Roasted Turkey Breast with Herbs

Ingredients:

- 2 pounds boneless, skinless turkey breast
- 1 tablespoon olive oil
- 2 tablespoons chopped fresh rosemary
- 1 tablespoon chopped fresh thyme
- 1 teaspoon garlic powder
- ½ teaspoon black pepper

Instructions:

1. Rub turkey with oil and seasonings. Place in a roasting pan.
2. Roast at 350°F for 50–60 minutes or until the thermometer reads 165°F. Rest before slicing.

Millet Pilaf with Greens and Pumpkin Seeds

Ingredients:

- 1 cup millet
- 2 cups low-sodium vegetable broth
- 2 cups chopped kale or spinach
- ¼ cup pumpkin seeds
- 1 tablespoon lemon juice
- 2 tablespoons olive oil

Instructions:

1. Rinse millet, add to pot with broth and bring to boil.
2. Reduce to simmer, cover, cook for 20 minutes; stir in greens for the last 5 minutes.
3. Fluff with fork; sprinkle pumpkin seeds and drizzle lemon and oil before serving.

Zucchini, Chickpea, and Tomato Casserole

Ingredients:

- 1 zucchini, diced
- 1 can (15 ounces) crushed tomatoes, drained
- 1 cup cooked chickpeas
- 1 red bell pepper, chopped
- 2 tablespoons olive oil
- 1 teaspoon dried basil

Instructions:

1. Sauté zucchini and bell pepper in olive oil until tender.
2. Layer in a baking dish with tomatoes, chickpeas, and basil.
3. Cover and bake at 375°F for 25 minutes.

Roasted Cauliflower with Turmeric

Ingredients:

- 1 large cauliflower, florets separated
- 2 tablespoons olive oil
- 1 teaspoon ground turmeric
- ½ teaspoon salt

Instructions:

1. Preheat the oven to 425°F. Toss cauliflower with oil, turmeric, and salt.
2. Roast 25 minutes, turning once.

Mediterranean Lentil Stew

Ingredients:

- 1 cup dry green or brown lentils
- 1 can (14 ounces) diced tomatoes
- 4 cups low-sodium vegetable broth
- 1 onion, chopped
- 1 cup chopped celery
- 1 cup chopped carrot
- 2 cloves garlic, minced
- 1 teaspoon cumin
- 2 tablespoons olive oil

Instructions:

1. Sauté onion, celery, carrot, and garlic in oil for 5 minutes. Add all remaining ingredients.
2. Simmer for 35 minutes, until the lentils are tender.

Maple-Baked Acorn Squash

Ingredients:

- 1 acorn squash, halved and seeded
- 2 teaspoons olive oil
- 1 tablespoon maple syrup or sugar-free syrup
- Pinch cinnamon

Instructions:

1. Preheat the oven to 400°F. Brush squash with oil, syrup, and cinnamon.
2. Place cut-side down on baking sheet; bake 35–40 minutes, until tender.

Zucchini Noodle Primavera

Ingredients:

- 4 zucchinis, spiralized or peeled into ribbons
- 1 red bell pepper, sliced
- 1 cup cherry tomatoes, halved
- 1 cup snow peas
- 2 tablespoons olive oil
- 1 tablespoon lemon juice

Instructions:

1. Sauté all vegetables in olive oil in a large skillet 5–6 minutes, add lemon juice; toss gently.

Herbed Lentil and Vegetable Patties

Ingredients:

- 1½ cups cooked lentils
- 1 potato, boiled and mashed
- 1 small carrot, grated
- 2 tablespoons flaxseed meal
- 1 teaspoon cumin
- 2 tablespoons chopped parsley

Instructions:

1. Mash all ingredients together; form 6 patties.
2. Pan-fry in olive oil over medium heat, 3 minutes per side.

Multi-Cooker and Slow-Cooker Recipe Adaptations

For those looking to conserve energy or prepare in advance, most of these recipes can be adapted for a multi-cooker (like an Instant Pot) or slow-cooker. **Here's how to convert:**

- **For stews, chilies, and lentil-based dishes:** Sauté any aromatics (onion, garlic, spices) in the pot, then add vegetables, legumes, and broth. Cook on high pressure for about 10–15 minutes, or in a slow cooker on low for 4–6 hours.
- **For roasts or one-pan meals:** Arrange components in the vessel as directed, drizzle with oil or sauce, and cook on low in a slow-cooker for 4–6 hours, or use the roast function in a multi-cooker.
- **Burgers and patties are best pan-cooked, as they benefit from a crisp exterior and gentle handling.** However, if standing at the stove is a challenge, you can also bake them on a parchment-lined baking sheet at 375°F for about 20 minutes, flipping halfway through. This hands-off approach maintains texture and ease of preparation.

- **For best results with all recipes, taste and adjust seasonings as needed, and feel free to swap in familiar herbs, spices, or vegetables according to personal preference and any dietary restrictions.** Remember to keep portions moderate and pair main dishes with one or two of the suggested sides for a well-rounded, anti-inflammatory dinner experience.

With these recipes and adaptations, dinnertime can remain a nourishing and pleasurable ritual for older adults managing neuropathy balancing flavor, comfort, and accessibility every evening.

Lifestyle Habits to Complement Your Neuropathy Nutrition Plan

When the kitchen has been tidied, the evening meal enjoyed, and perhaps your favorite show is winding down, what happens next is quietly powerful for anyone managing neuropathy. Small daily actions—how you move, care for your feet, wind down for sleep, drink water, and expose yourself to sunlight—hold surprising leverage over nerve pain, balance, and day-to-day comfort. While nutrition is a foundational pillar, evidence suggests its benefits multiply when woven with practical lifestyle habits designed specifically for older adults and their unique needs.

Let's walk through what an integrated day might look like for a senior seeking not just fewer neuropathy symptoms, but a greater sense of capability and rhythm. Rather than viewing each habit in isolation, consider how sensory-friendly movement, foot care, restorative rest, hydration, and gentle sunlight complement what's on your plate. Each approach below is grounded in research and adapted for varying mobility, age-related limitations, and the fluctuating reality of living with peripheral neuropathy.

Sensory-Safe Movement and Balance: Nerve-Supportive Activity at Home

Daily movement is not just about burning calories or building muscle. For older adults with neuropathy, regular, gentle activity helps maintain microcirculation which delivers oxygen to peripheral nerves, stabilizes blood sugar, improves balance, and counteracts the muscle weakness or unsteadiness that nerve damage often brings. What's crucial is exercising in ways that are safe for feet and joints, respect altered sensation, and can be adapted for different activity levels or mobility aids.

Here's a sample home routine, crafted for safety and flexibility:

1. **Marching in Place, Seated or Standing**

If balance is a concern, sit toward the front edge of a sturdy chair, hold onto the sides, and gently lift your knees one at a time, "marching" for 1–2 minutes. If standing is comfortable, hold the back of a chair or kitchen counter for support. This movement gets blood flowing to the lower legs and feet without excessive strain.

2. **Side Leg Lifts**

Standing beside a table or counter for support, lift one leg to the side as far as comfortable, lower, then switch. Repeat 8–12 times per side. The motion engages hip muscles and helps with lateral stability—key for preventing falls.

3. **Gentle Toe and Heel Raises**

Holding a support, come up gently onto your toes, lower, then rock back onto your heels. Repeat 10 times. This strengthens ankle muscles and supports circulation in the feet.

4. **Balancing "Tandem Stand"**

Stand with one foot directly in front of the other, heel to toe. Use a countertop or sturdy chair for support. Try to hold for 10 seconds; switch feet. Even brief holds help "re-train" the brain and body for steadier walking.

5. **Seated Overhead Arm Stretch**

In a chair, raise both arms overhead, reaching upward and gently stretching the sides. Hold for several breaths. This not only increases shoulder mobility but signals the body to wake up gently.

The routine can be performed once or twice daily, with all movements tailored for comfort. Before beginning any new exercise regimen, check with your doctor or physical therapist, especially if you experience dizziness, marked numbness, or have a history of falls. All props (chairs, non-slip mats, supportive shoes) should be close at hand for stability.

Safety adaptations include:

- Practicing in a clutter-free space free of trip hazards.
- Using a walker or cane if helpful.
- Working with a caregiver or family member nearby for reassurance, especially early on.
- Adjusting repetitions or resting as needed when fatigue, pain, or unsteadiness arise.

By focusing less on "how much" and more on "how safely" you move, you're doing what matters most for nerve integrity and injury prevention.

Gentle Stretching, Foot Care, and Self-Massage: Preventing Problems Before They Begin

Consistent attention to your feet and lower legs is as important as your nutrition plan. Stretching, paired with daily foot care, helps relax tight muscles, encourages circulation, and prevents the stiffness or pressure points that can escalate into sores or infection for those with reduced sensation.

A simple evening protocol:

- **Calf Stretch (Seated or Standing):** Place both hands on a wall, step one foot back, and gently press the heel into the floor. Hold for 20–30 seconds per side. If unsteady standing, loop a towel under your foot (while seated) and gently pull toward you to stretch the calf.
- **Ankle Circles:** While sitting, extend one leg and slowly rotate the ankle 10 times in each direction. Repeat for the other leg.
- **Toe Spread and Squeeze:** Spread your toes wide, hold for five seconds, then press them together. Repeat 10–12 times. This helps keep tiny foot muscles active and alert.

For foot care:

- **Inspect both feet daily under good lighting.** Use a mirror for hard-to-see areas. Looking for blisters, redness, cuts, swelling, or changes in skin color addressing problems early reduces the risk of severe complications.

- **Wash feet in lukewarm (not hot) water, pat dry, and moisturize the tops and bottoms.** Keep skin between the toes dry to prevent fungal growth.
- **Trim toenails straight across, not too short, and file any rough edges gently.** If nails are thick or hard to cut, a podiatrist can help avoid injury.

Gentle massage (using lotion or oil) after washing can help reduce stiffness, soothe nerve endings, and improve circulation without vigorous pressure. Start with light strokes on the soles and tops of your feet, moving up to the ankles and lower calves. Even a brief, mindful massage can calm nerve signals and foster a sense of relaxation before bed.

If you notice new numbness, persistent sores, or any wounds that do not heal, communicate promptly with your healthcare provider.

Sleep Hygiene to Ease Neuropathy Discomfort and Night Pain

For many seniors, neuropathy-related discomfort intensifies at night making sleep feel just beyond reach. Yet, good sleep is essential for pain tolerance, nerve repair, stable mood, and immune function. Adapting your sleep routines to address pain and sensory disturbances can support both physical healing and day-to-day optimism.

Consider this sequence for better nighttime comfort:

- **Establish a Consistent Sleep and Wake Schedule:** Go to bed and rise at the same time daily, even on weekends. This regularity helps regulate your circadian rhythm, making it easier to fall and stay asleep.
- **Create a Predictable Wind-Down Routine:** Slow the pace 60 minutes before bedtime. This could include listening to calm music, gentle stretching, or reading something enjoyable (aim for comfort, not stimulation).
- **Assess Your Sleep Environment:** Choose a supportive mattress and consider an extra pillow to elevate your legs, which may reduce tingling or burning sensations. Soft, loose bedding helps prevent pressure on sensitive feet or hands.
- **Temperature and Light:** Keep your room cool and dark. A lightweight blanket can be comforting, but avoid heavy covers on affected limbs.
- **Addressing Physical Discomfort:** Use a warm (not hot) water bottle on feet or hands if cold, or a cool pack if burning pain is prominent. Always protect your skin with a towel and check that you don't have impaired sensation before applying temperature-based comfort.
- **Pre-Bedtime Nutrition:** Avoid large, heavy meals and limit fluid intake an hour before bed to reduce trips to the restroom. Choose small portions of anti-inflammatory snacks if hungry Greek yogurt, a banana, or a handful of walnuts are options that align with nerve-supporting nutrition.

If pain spikes interrupt sleep, brief relaxation techniques such as slow breathing, focusing on a calming memory, or gentle self-massage may encourage your body back to rest. Discuss severe or persistent nighttime pain with your medical team to ensure all avenues of care (including pain management and medication timing) have been considered.

Hydration and Light Exposure: Orchestrating Daytime Energy and Symptom Calm

Fluid status and exposure to daylight both influence nerve function, meal metabolism, and alertness for older adults. Dehydration can worsen sensations of tingling, amplify fatigue, and disrupt blood sugar control particularly critical for seniors with diabetic neuropathy or common age-related kidney changes.

Here's how to structure hydration and light for maximum benefit:

- **Begin your morning with a glass of water**—ideally within 30 minutes of waking and before breakfast. This prepares your nervous system and digestive tract for the day's activity.
- **Aim to drink modest amounts of water throughout the day, pairing each meal with 4–8 ounces (half to one cup).** Small, regular sips are easier to manage than large gulps and reduce the risk of nighttime bathroom visits.
- **Limit caffeinated beverages and avoid sugary drinks, as both can spike or drop blood sugar and increase dehydration risk.** Moderate intake of herbal teas or diluted 100% fruit juices can add variety.

Aligning your day with natural light helps regulate circadian rhythms and supports better sleep at night. After breakfast or morning movement, spend 15–30 minutes by a window, on a porch, or in your yard to let your eyes and skin absorb daylight. If venturing outside isn't possible, sit in brightly lit areas indoors and open window coverings to maximize indirect sunlight.

Light exposure is especially relevant to seniors managing both neuropathy and seasonal affective shifts, as it can elevate mood and reset the body's natural sleep-wake cues. Avoid bright screens and harsh lighting in the hour before bed, as "blue light" exposure can signal your brain that it's still daytime, delaying sleep onset and aggravating night-time nerve symptoms.

Integrating Nutrition, Movement, and Rest: A Practical Lifestyle Support Framework

Rather than treating each pillar, food, movement, rest as isolated boxes on a to-do list, the strongest improvements emerge when they form a rhythm across your week. Below is an integrated schedule that models how an anti-inflammatory eating plan harmonizes with movement, hydration, and restorative routines. Adapt the timing and sequencing to suit your needs, energy fluctuations, and medical instructions:

A Sample Daily Routine

Morning

- **Upon waking:** Drink a glass of water. Open curtains or step onto a balcony for 15 minutes of daylight exposure, if possible.

- **After breakfast:** Complete a sensory-safe movement routine (marching, balance, stretches as outlined above).
- **Late morning:** Enjoy a low-glycemic snack if needed, and consider a brief walk inside your home or along a safe path.

Midday

- **Lunch:** Prioritize protein, whole grains, and colorful vegetables for ongoing energy. Pair with water or an herbal infusion.
- **After lunch:** Gentle stretching or a 5-minute walk. Inspect feet for pressure spots or footwear concerns.

Afternoon

- **Hydrate steadily with water or tea.** Change sitting positions regularly to keep blood moving and avoid stiffness.
- **If fatigued, try a 15–20 minute rest or calming activity rather than a long nap,** supporting healthy nighttime sleep.

Evening

- **Dinner:** Focus on anti-inflammatory recipes rich in fiber, lean protein, and healthy fats.
- **After dinner:** Wind-down with quiet reading, music, or light conversation. Avoid heavy exercise or large meals after 7 pm.
- **Sleep hygiene:** Begin your wind-down routine an hour before bed. Check feet one final time and apply gentle massage or moisturize as desired.

Weekly Planning

- **Combine grocery shopping with movement** (walking the aisles or standing while prepping food counts, too).

- **If energy is low, batch-cook on days when you feel strongest;** freeze meals for easier access later in the week.
- **Set reminders** for hydration, foot inspection, and movement breaks using alarms or visual cues.
- Plan at least one longer walk or structured movement session per week, weather and safety permitting.

By integrating these daily touchpoints, you avoid the all-or-nothing cycle that can be discouraging or unsustainable. Each element whether a glass of water, a gentle toe circle, or a 10-minute rest—contributes to a cumulative, positive effect on nerve health and symptom management.

Troubleshooting and Adjusting Your Routine

Even the best routines will sometimes falter, maybe a poor night's sleep, extra fatigue, or an unexpected symptom flare makes full participation challenging. Expect and normalize these shifts, focusing on adapting rather than abandoning your supportive rhythm.

On low energy days:

- Prioritize hydration, minimal movement (such as seated stretches), and small foot inspections.
- Choose easier meals you've prepped in advance or simple, anti-inflammatory snacks.
- Communicate changes in symptoms, sleep, or comfort to a family member, caregiver, or health provider if you notice escalating pain, new numbness, or sores that do not heal.

Seniors prone to low motivation or living alone may benefit from:

- Setting up scheduled phone check-ins with a friend for shared movement or meal times.
- Posting your simplified routine on the fridge for visual reinforcement.
- Using music or radio as cues to begin movement, mealtime, or stretching.

Review your routines biweekly or monthly: Are pain patterns improving? Do meals feel easier to prepare? Is balance more stable during daily activities? Adjust frequency, timing, or types of activities as needed, or consult your healthcare team for further adaptations.

The science of nerve health confirms that symptom relief is more than a one-dimensional solution. Nutrition, while critical, is most effective when embedded within a fabric of movement, hydration, circadian rhythm tuning, and proactive self-care. This synergy not only supports metabolic function and reduces inflammation, but also addresses the daily practical realities of painful nights, unpredictable numbness, and the risk of falls or ulcers that older adults with neuropathy may face.

This lifestyle framework invites you to build small, sustainable habits rather than chase unachievable standards. Consistency, adaptation, and kindness to yourself are the paramount tools, ensuring that the gains made in anti-inflammatory eating translate into comfort, safety, and confidence in everyday life.

Keep this foundation as you progress regardless of new recipes or updated protocols. Every step, stretch, restful night, and glass of water is an act of support for your nerves and your well-being.

Symptom Tracking, Adjustment, and Long-Term Maintenance

Between carefully preparing meals and settling into supportive daily routines, living with neuropathy as an older adult means tuning into your body's signals, tracking progress and gently adjusting both food and lifestyle as needed. This ongoing process helps ensure that improvements last, setbacks are caught early, and clinicians remain fully informed partners in your care. While nutrition and lifestyle changes can lay a strong foundation, a smart maintenance plan translates that initial momentum into real, day-to-day comfort and safety.

Rather than relying on memory or trial and error, the combination of simple symptom logging, structured adjustments, and proactive maintenance offers a path forward that is practical, empowering, and firmly grounded in current science. Let's explore in detail how to make tracking, tweaking, and sustaining progress both realistic and rewarding.

Building Your Symptom and Nutrition Log

When it comes to managing neuropathy, subjective impressions like "I think my feet feel better this week" are valuable, but structured records are even more powerful. A basic log serves several purposes at once: it helps you notice patterns, makes communication with healthcare providers more precise, and allows for adjustments based on real evidence rather than guesswork. For many older adults, simple consistency wins over high-tech tools.

Begin with a template that covers the following categories for each day:

Sample Log Entry:

- **Date:** April 5
- **Meals:** Oatmeal + berries (breakfast); lentil soup (lunch); chicken, sweet potato, broccoli (dinner); apple (snack)
- **Hydration:** ~6 cups water + 1 herbal tea
- **Activity:** 10-min walk after breakfast, chair stretches in afternoon
- **Symptoms:** Numbness (feet, 3/10 AM, 4/10 PM); mild tingling (fingers, evening); no sores
- **Mood/Energy:** Steady, a little low energy after lunch
- **Sleep:** 7.5 hours, woke once (foot discomfort)
- **Meds:** No changes
- **Notes:** Feet checked, no new red spots

Most find that jotting quick notes at meal times and before bed takes less than five minutes. Some prefer making check marks or using a weekly grid layout, especially if writing is tiring. If vision or dexterity is limited, voice-recording on a smartphone or having a caregiver help fill out the log works just as well.

This "living record" keeps daily management grounded in reality and builds a detailed timeline to share with your doctor, dietitian, or specialist.

Refining Your Routine: Adjustment Based on Patterns

No two neuropathy experiences follow the exact same course, so your log supports both predictability and necessary adaptation. After several days or weeks, look for the following response trends:

- Symptom improvement on days after anti-inflammatory meals or more balanced hydration
- Setbacks or worsened numbness after consuming processed foods, excess sugar, or salt
- Sleep disruptions tied to heavier evening meals or late-night snacking
- Activity or movement levels that seem to ease or aggravate symptoms
- Reactions to new supplements, vitamins, or medications

A few guiding rules help you adjust your plan:

1. If you observe noted improvements in pain or energy after specific meal patterns such as increased leafy greens, healthy fats, or omega-3-rich foods aim to maintain or repeat those meals through the week.
2. Should a particular food trigger increased tingling, pain, or gastrointestinal discomfort, consider removing it temporarily and monitoring symptom changes over the next two weeks.
3. When physical activity leads to soreness or balance issues, reduce the intensity or switch from standing to seated exercises. Conversely, gentle daily movement often leads to improved comfort over several consecutive days.

4. Persistent fatigue or lower-than-expected improvement may prompt adjustments in hydration, rest timing, or meal portion size, rather than drastic food eliminations.
5. Track any changes introduced by healthcare providers (new medication, supplement regimen) for at least a week. Make note of positive or negative symptom changes.

Remember that meaningful improvements in nerve function are gradual; dietary shifts may bring energy stabilization and some symptom relief within two to four weeks, but greater nerve benefits are gradual and take patience. An integrative approach combining food, activity, and clinical treatments—produces the best long-term results. Quick changes, especially in older adults, can stress the system or mask progress.

Safety Signals: When to Involve Your Physician

Proactive tracking equips you to celebrate gains, but just as importantly, it helps you recognize when it's time to seek medical input, rather than relying solely on lifestyle shifts. **The following are clear indicators for prompt consultation:**

- New or rapidly worsening numbness, tingling, or weakness in the feet, hands, or other areas
- Persistent foot or skin injuries that do not heal or show signs of infection (redness, swelling, discharge)
- Sudden changes in digestion (such as severe constipation or diarrhea), urination, or bladder control

- Significant drops in blood pressure or frequent dizziness (especially in people managing diabetes or multiple medications)
- New or severe burning pain, especially if interfering with sleep or daily activity
- Rapid weight loss without intent, or unexplained changes in appetite

If improvements plateau despite consistent efforts, or if new symptoms appear, your nutrition plan may need to be adjusted in partnership with a healthcare professional to prevent further complications. Early identification and professional treatment is essential to avoid worsening nerve damage. Diet, while supportive, does not replace clinical care.

Routine periodic reviews with a clinician are especially critical for older adults with complex conditions or those taking multiple medications. Sharing your symptom and nutrition log during visits informs safer, more effective medical adjustments and avoids the risks of uncoordinated changes at home.

Long-Term Maintenance: Sustaining Progress After the 28-Day Recovery Plan

The conclusion of the structured 28-Day Neuropathy Protocol does not mark the end of your journey but the beginning of a sustainable pattern. Transitioning from an "intensive" to a "steady state" means maintaining gains without burnout. **Four pillars support ongoing maintenance:**

1. **Rotating Recipes and Food Choices:**

Return to the core meal templates from the recovery plan, selecting at least two to three recipes each for breakfast, lunch, and dinner to cycle throughout the month. Vary vegetables, grains, and proteins seasonally to avoid monotony and encourage a broader spectrum of micronutrients. Batch-cooking or freezing four-serving portions helps manage low-energy days.

2. **Scheduling Regular Activity Renewal:**

Plan for at least one structured movement session daily, adapted for your abilities. Combine gentle stretches and balance exercises with more enjoyable activities (gardening, walking with a friend, or mild chair yoga) to keep engagement high. Twice a month, revisit new exercise ideas or review routines with a physical therapist when possible.

3. **Ongoing Hydration and Snack Management:**

Continue the pattern of scheduled water intake (with each meal and between) and choose snack options aligned with anti-inflammatory principles: nuts, Greek yogurt, berries, or pre-cut vegetables. Monitor any changes needed for dental, swallowing, or digestive difficulties, adjusting snack texture and size as your needs evolve.

4. **Regular Symptom and Meal Review:**

Each month, review the symptom and nutrition log for shifts in patterns, new foods added, or activity changes. Share this periodic review with a healthcare provider either in person or remotely to fine-tune the maintenance plan.

Sustaining progress is rarely about perfection. Instead, it's the process of consistent self-awareness, strategic substitutions, and adapting supportive routines that fit with energy, motivation, and changing medical conditions in later life.

Potential Medication-Nutrition Interactions: Staying Safe and Informed

Many older adults with neuropathy may be prescribed medications for conditions such as diabetes, high cholesterol, high blood pressure, or nerve pain—sometimes several at the same time. Because nutrition and medications can interact in important ways, regularly reviewing these combinations with a healthcare provider is recommended.

Common interactions relevant to seniors with neuropathy include:

- **Metformin (used for diabetes) and reduced vitamin B12 absorption:** Long-term use can cause B12 deficiency, increasing the risk of worsening neuropathy. Routine monitoring and, when necessary, supplementation is key.
- **Statins (for cholesterol) and muscle or nerve effects:** Some statins, in combination with low CoQ10 from diet, can exacerbate muscle pain or weakness.
- **Diuretics (often prescribed for blood pressure):** May deplete potassium, magnesium, or sodium, leading to cramps, fatigue, or worsened neuropathic symptoms.

- **Certain antibiotics or antifungals:** May interact with supplements or specific foods—always check with your pharmacist when starting a new prescription.
- **Alcohol and sedating medications:** These can interact negatively and impair balance, further increasing the risk of falls or accidents in individuals with neuropathy.

Even familiar over-the-counter supplements, such as B vitamins or magnesium, can interact with prescription drugs in unexpected ways, sometimes reducing drug efficacy or triggering side effects. For example, some antacid medications can decrease the absorption of vitamin B12 or magnesium, further complicating nerve health if unmanaged.

Because polypharmacy is common and interactions are so individualized, consult a healthcare professional or a registered dietitian before making significant dietary changes or introducing new supplements.

Sustaining gains after the initial recovery protocol calls for more than just willpower or rigid routines. It's an ongoing loop: observe, adjust, and renew. The daily log fosters attentiveness; gentle modifications address both setbacks and successes. Active collaboration with your healthcare team guards against silent complications and helps you match your lifestyle with your medications and changing circumstances.

With each entry in your log, every low-sodium or antioxidant-rich meal, and each day that includes safe movement and hydration, you reinforce the gains made during your recovery plan. The ultimate long-term success lies in flexible persistence, an approach where symptom tracking and informed adjustment empower you to face the unpredictable ups and downs of living with neuropathy.

This cycle of observation, careful tweaking, timely consultation, and regular renewal creates a robust foundation for maintaining nerve health and minimizing pain. Your personal observations and the insights from clinicians together point the way to a better quality of life rooted not in "cures," but in confidence, safety, and well-supported self-care.

Conclusion

Looking back at the nutrition strategies, lifestyle adjustments, and self-tracking methods described in this guide, one central message stands out: supporting nerve health as an older adult isn't about making quick changes, but about working steadily with your body, your care team, and the daily routines you choose. The choices you make about food, movement, rest, and self-monitoring create a flexible system that can adapt to your changing needs, while still being structured enough to help you make real progress, even when life gets tough.

By now, you have the basics: an understanding of the common causes and types of neuropathy in seniors, simple ways to build anti-inflammatory meals, a phased 28-day recovery plan, and a customizable maintenance routine. Each part is meant to help you figure out what helps or bothers your symptoms, instead of forcing one "right" way to eat or live. This respect for your individual needs is important, because everyone's path to comfort and stability looks a little different especially later in life.

Taking action like swapping in a few nerve-friendly breakfasts, trying gentle stretches, or keeping a daily log might seem like a small step. But research and real-life experience show that making steady, thoughtful choices often leads to better energy, mood, and symptom relief within weeks for many seniors with neuropathy. Some days you'll notice clear progress; other days might bring new challenges or questions. By observing and adjusting as you go, lasting comfort becomes more possible.

No guide or plan, no matter how thorough, can replace your doctor's expertise especially if your symptoms suddenly change or new issues come up. Medical care is still essential for finding the causes, checking medications, and helping with more complicated decisions. But the simple, everyday care you give yourself through nutrition, hydration, movement, and gentle check-ins can lighten the load of neuropathy, help prevent complications, and even make your medical appointments more effective.

Building your own routine for nerve comfort means weaving helpful habits into your everyday life. This could mean rotating favorite recipes to keep things interesting, adjusting your approach if symptoms stick around, and always feeling comfortable to ask questions or update those involved in your care. Even when progress is slow, tracking, reflecting, and working together help you gain more clarity and control.

For older adults, good nutrition and self-care routines do more than just support health—they can bring back a sense of independence and enjoyment to daily life, which chronic pain or discomfort often takes away. Making a nourishing meal, taking a safe walk with a friend, or simply waking up feeling a bit better can be ways to care for yourself and celebrate your own resilience.

As you move forward, try to stay curious. Use your log not just to keep records, but to spark conversations. Let your meals show both what's good for your nerves and what you enjoy eating. Reach out to your care team quickly if things change or you have questions, and invite friends or family to join in when it feels right. This process isn't about being perfect; it's about finding a gentler, steadier way to care for yourself day by day, season by season.

Managing neuropathy is a personal experience, but with the help and structure in these chapters, each step you take is proof of your commitment and ability. Your actions truly can support better nerve health, comfort, and vitality not just for a moment, but through the thoughtful choices you make every day.

FAQs

Which foods most reliably worsen or improve neuropathy symptoms in seniors?

Certain foods promote nerve health, while others can aggravate symptoms. *Improving* foods include whole grains, legumes, nuts, seeds, non-starchy vegetables, and most fruits—foods high in fiber, vitamins, minerals, and essential fatty acids. These support balanced blood sugar and provide key nutrients for nerve repair and function. Anti-inflammatory choices like leafy greens, berries, fatty fish, nuts, turmeric, and ginger also support nerve health and may ease symptoms.

Foods that *worsen* symptoms include those made with refined flour (white bread, pasta, pastries), sugary snacks, fried foods, processed items, and too much alcohol. These promote inflammation and blood sugar swings, which can intensify nerve pain. Some artificial sweeteners, such as aspartame, saccharin, and sucralose, may also increase pain or sensitivity in some individuals. For people with gluten intolerance or celiac disease, gluten-containing grains can further aggravate nerve issues.

How should supplements like B12, magnesium, or alpha-lipoic acid be used safely with medications?

Older adults with neuropathy often have deficiencies in B vitamins—especially B1, B6, and B12—or magnesium, all important for nerve health. While it is safest to meet needs through food, supplements may be required if bloodwork or restrictions prevent adequate intake. Supplements should only be taken with a physician's guidance: your doctor can recommend appropriate doses, test your levels, and check for interactions with other medications.

This protects against excessive intake and dangerous drug-nutrient interactions. Alpha-lipoic acid, an antioxidant, is sometimes used as an adjunct for neuropathy, but should only be added in consultation with your care team. Do not change doses or add new supplements without your physician's approval, as some nutrients can interfere with blood thinners, heart, or diabetes medications. Safe supplementation requires close coordination of your nutrition plan and medications.

What are common signs that nerve pain is getting worse or needs medical attention?

Neuropathy symptoms can fluctuate, but certain changes require prompt attention. Persistent or increasing pain, spreading numbness, tingling, or new weakness in your hands or feet call for medical evaluation. So do wounds on your feet that won't heal, sudden balance problems, or new difficulties with digestion, urination, or sexual function.

While diet can help diminish symptoms and prevent further progression, it cannot reverse advanced nerve injury. Worsening or new symptoms need timely medical follow-up to prevent complications and adjust treatment.

How can recipes be adjusted for chewing, swallowing, or digestive problems common in older adults?

For chewing or swallowing problems, choose soft foods: soups, stews, smoothies, and steamed or mashed vegetables are easier to eat. Pureeing or finely chopping meals reduces choking risk. If digestion is slowed or constipation is present, slowly increase fiber using oats, flaxseed, or soft-cooked beans and ensure good hydration.

Use thickening agents like mashed avocado or yogurt for easier swallowing. For sensitive digestion, stick to mild spices and avoid greasy dishes. Serve meals warm—not hot—and offer smaller, more frequent portions.

What kitchen tools or strategies help seniors with limited grip or vision?

Adapting your kitchen can make meal prep easier. Use utensils with ergonomic, non-slip handles. Electric jar openers, food processors, and adaptive cutting boards reduce hand strain. Choose color-contrasting mats and plates to enhance visibility, and use non-slip mats under work surfaces.

Portion-controlled scoops, measuring cups with large markings, and finger guards make cooking safer. Appliances like slow cookers, rice cookers, and single-touch gadgets can save energy and build confidence. Pre-cut or pre-portioned ingredients, when affordable, also simplify preparation.

How soon might symptom changes appear with this protocol, and what's realistic for older adults?

Some symptom relief—like more stable energy, improved blood sugar, or less fatigue—may appear in two to four weeks after dietary changes. More significant nerve function improvements generally take months and are gradual. In older adults, goals are often to restore nutrients, stabilize glucose, and reduce symptom severity; complete reversal of symptoms is uncommon. Continuing the recommended habits alongside prescribed treatment brings the best results.

What resources aid with menu planning and shopping when independence is reduced?

If shopping or meal planning is difficult, resources like print-friendly food lists, menu templates, and shopping guides (such as those found in this book) can help. Family or caregivers can assist with planning and shopping. Many retailers offer online ordering with curbside pickup or home delivery for those with mobility or stamina challenges. Community and senior centers may provide condition-specific meal deliveries. When possible, batch cooking or sharing prep with others promotes variety and food safety.

By making small daily changes balancing nutrition, adapting kitchen tools, and monitoring symptoms older adults with neuropathy can maintain greater comfort and independence, working closely with caregivers and medical teams.

References and Helpful Links

ARĂMESCU, A.. Sexual dysfunctions in diabetic neuropathy. https://doi.org/10.37072/jcs.2022.02.03

Bowsher, D.. (1999). The lifetime occurrence of Herpes zoster and prevalence of post-herpetic neuralgia: A retrospective survey in an elderly population. *European Journal of Pain*. https://doi.org/10.1016/s1090-3801(99)90015-0

Minerd, M.. What You Don't Know Can Still Harm You. https://doi.org/10.5840/ncbq202323450

Humphries, T., Kushalnagar, P., Mathur, G. et al.. Support for parents of deaf children: Common questions and informed, evidence-based answers. https://doi.org/10.1016/j.ijporl.2018.12.036

Calder, P.. Omega-3 fatty acids and inflammatory processes: from molecules to man. https://doi.org/10.1042/bst20160474

Ziegler, D.. Diabetic Peripheral and Autonomic Neuropathy. https://doi.org/10.1002/9781118924853.ch40

Shivappa, N., Bosetti, C., Zucchetto, A. et al.. Dietary inflammatory index and risk of pancreatic cancer in an Italian case–control study. https://doi.org/10.1017/s0007114514003626

Hernandez-Cardoso, G., Amador-Medina, L., Gutierrez-Torres, G. et al.. (2022). Terahertz imaging demonstrates its diagnostic potential and reveals a relationship between cutaneous dehydration and neuropathy for diabetic foot syndrome patients. *Scientific Reports*. https://doi.org/10.1038/s41598-022-06996-w

Zhou, X., Shi, H., Zhu, S. et al.. Effects of vitamin E and vitamin C on male infertility: a meta-analysis. https://doi.org/10.1007/s11255-022-03237-x

Unknown Author. (2017). Effects of a long-term lifestyle modification programme on peripheral neuropathy in overweight or obese adults with type 2 diabetes: the Look AHEAD study. *Diabetologia*. https://doi.org/10.1007/s00125-017-4253-z

Mold, J., Vesely, S., Keyl, B. et al.. (2004). The Prevalence, Predictors, and Consequences of Peripheral Sensory Neuropathy in Older Patients. *The Journal of the American Board of Family Medicine*. https://doi.org/10.3122/jabfm.17.5.309

www.ingramcontent.com/pod-product-compliance
Lightning Source LLC
LaVergne TN
LVHW010724061126
851857LV00014B/1329